IKIGAI

Develop Your Areas of Success, Ikigai Strategy

(The Secret to Understanding Your Purpose for a Fulfilling Life)

Howard Moffett

Published By Howard Moffett

Howard Moffett

IKIGAI: Develop Your Areas of Success, Ikigai Strategy (The Secret to Understanding Your Purpose for a Fulfilling Life)

ISBN 978-1-77485-411-2

Legal & Disclaimer

The information contained in this book is not designed to replace or take the place of any form of medicine or professional medical advice. The information in this book has been provided for educational and entertainment purposes only.

The information contained in this book has been compiled from sources deemed reliable, and it is accurate to the best of the Author's knowledge; however, the Author cannot guarantee its accuracy and validity and cannot be held liable for any errors or omissions. Changes are periodically made to this book. You must consult your doctor or get professional medical advice before using any of the suggested remedies, techniques, or information in this book.

Upon using the information contained in this book, you agree to hold harmless the Author from and against any damages, costs, and expenses, including any legal fees potentially resulting from the application of any of the information provided by this guide. This disclaimer applies to any damages or injury caused by the use and application, whether directly or

TABLE OF CONTENTS

INTRODUCTION 1

CHAPTER 1: IKIGAI MEANINGS IN JAPANESE 7

CHAPTER 2: FINDING YOUR WAY 23

CHAPTER 3: FOUR REGIONS OF THE IKIGAI...................... 46

CHAPTER 4: PHYSICAL TRAINING TO UNLOCK YOUR IKIGAI
.... 66

CHAPTER 5: ANTIAGING SECRETS 92

CHAPTER 6: WHAT'S YOUR IGAI? 117

CHAPTER 7: THE VENN DIAGRAM WITH THE PURPOSE.. 127

CHAPTER 8: FOUR FEELINGS THAT INFLUENCE THE COURSE
OF YOUR IKIGAI DISCOVERY JOURNEY 144

CHAPTER 9: BUSINESS MODEL OF MAKING SOCIETY HAPPY
.... 152

CHAPTER 10: IKIGAI AND HEALTH 163

CONCLUSION... 177

Introduction

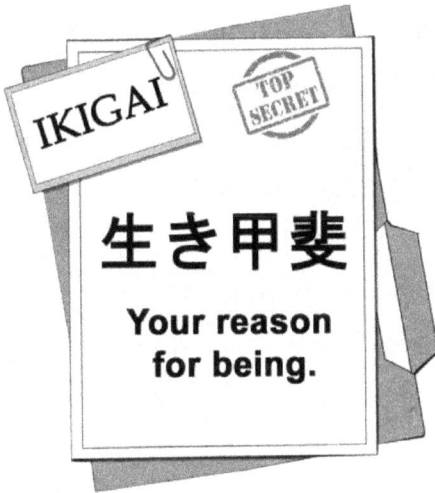

In the past, customs stipulated that one generation followed one another in the decision of what to do. You followed in the footsteps of your parents and followed their example. However, towards the close of the century, things began to change.

In the 1980s, a perfect career was believed to be all about following the money. Everyone was searching for opportunities to invest in the latest trend and create huge fortunes. In the 1990s the emphasis changed and was now about following your interests. The issue in this is, when we're young, our passions can be very limited. Rockstar actors, sportspersons artists, etc. We'll be honest, only a small percentage of people actually succeed in these fields, and so simply following our passions often isn't enough to be successful by itself. Since the turn of the millennium there has been a major shift in thinking and more recently , the emphasis has been on doing work that is considered important and actually aids others. However, this isn't enough. There are so many choices. How do you decide what you should pick? This is the point where Ikigai is a great help. It could be helpful if:

Are you looking to accomplish something that gives you genuine satisfaction, happiness and a feeling of accomplishment

If you feel that you're not on the right path in your life?

* Are you tired of the need to wake up and get ready for work every day

* Hate your job

* Do you have dreams that aren't realized of living a more fulfilling life

* Are you looking to contribute to the world and aid others in any way?

Do you want to find an ardent passion for what you're doing in your life

Have you ever sitting on a bus , train, or in the subway, and you just stared at the other passengers? I've certainly been there. I'm curious about their lives as well as how they make a living, and whether they're happy. I believe that we all have the right to be happy and beyond our relationships, our work life has the greatest influence on this.

The Pew Research Centre in Washington D.C. In the Pew Research Centre in Washington D.C., it was revealed from a study that more than 30 percent of Americans were dissatisfied with their work. A majority of them said that their job was just to make ends meet. Although you may enjoy the work you do today, things might alter in the near future. It has been observed that as we age the way we think about our goals shift. If you are in an intense and lucrative job that demands lots of motivation and energy, in time, you'll become exhausted. What is the cost of being in a stressful environment? A premature death.

A lot of us are employed in large cities, in which just getting to work is stressful. When we surveyed people on a daily basis, it was the commute that people said they resent most about their job.

In time the most important thing to us is how we live our lives. As we get older, we develop new passions. As we grow older we tend to be ambitious. We imagine an excellent job, a large home, or a luxurious automobile. For some, these fantasies can be realized however for the vast majority of us, they're just ever fantasies. Reality bites , and most of the time, we find ourselves in work that we've never would have wanted to do or were intended to be temporary because we must pay the endless bills. When we reach a certain point, we are dissatisfied with our lives and begin to seek satisfaction. It could happen in a variety of ways, from eating too much to changing relationships.

Instead of bringing joy, these changes only bring new challenges. It's not really a matter of how we act. Happiness and fulfillment seem to be just beyond our reach.

What do you think Ikigai assist you? Ikigai helps you think about things from a new perspective or helps you to evaluate the things that are important to you. It prompts you to think about different things that you may not have considered before. It could open the door to a new world in which satisfaction and happiness is possible. All you need to do is transform the door into a window and then walk through. It's true that life isn't that long. Aren't we entitled to happiness and to live life to the fullest?

Chapter 1: Ikigai Meanings In Japanese

For many English natives, ikigai is detected and is spoken in three syllables. It is however, ikigai has four syllables according to the Japanese hiragana alphabet , below, and it is pronounced (Ee-Kee-Ga-Ee):

*Japanese Hiragana

*Ikigai Written In Japanese Kanji

In a literal sense"iki" means "life alive" and Kai (pronounced as gai in the context of this) can be translated to mean "reason worthiness efficient; fruitful." Concerning kai, it is important to note that it has a strong association with an issue. The most common assertion is that it is a result of the desire to succeed. It is therefore a valuable part of anyone's life, and requires the same amount of effort to achieve it. So the literal translation may not give you the knowledge you require to comprehend what the meaning of the phrase is and the implications for you. In the end there's a myriad of transcreations which are exact:

*Reason To Take Measure

*The Meaning Of Life

*Reason for Being

*The What is the meaning Of Life

*Reason To Wake Up In The Morning Or Upon Appearing In To Go to

What makes life price living?

The Issue You Have To Live For

*Happiness Of Being

*A Raison D'etre

*And Thus *And Therefore...

Are There Benefits to Ikigai?

For many, I am included in their space, they are frequently when we wake up, anxious about the day ahead. We are prone to lie on our backs for just a minute or two, reluctant to get started. We are sick of the seemingly mundane activities that we do in our daily lives called the"stuff" and we want to let ourselves become an in a closed-off animal that has to be cared for.

When we're feeling down, we have an urge to go on the routine of our lives and not pay attention, only conscious of the lack of enjoyment in the things we have to deal with. From day in to time out, reception or at work there is nothing that changes. We don't really enjoy the day, we are more likely to create our own day. At night, when we are prone to close our eyes at night, we're likely to be thinking about the awful day we'll face the next day. It's obvious that there's a better method.

Let's consider it, but ikigai can help you in the pursuit of happiness. Imagine being awestruck by the sensation of being energized especially on mornings on Mondays. But how nice would it be nice to know that the day ahead might be the same for you every day? That's what ikigai will do for you. It gives you the drive you need to enjoy life the way you'd like to live it. It's filled with enthusiasm. Be a part of your passions everyday and you'll certain be enthralled to keep going for a second time and more the next day, and the following day. Take a sip of ikigai and finish your speech saying, "Today was a good day. I'm alive today."

Motivation and Happiness

Let's take a look However, ikigai will assist you in your quest for happiness. Imagine getting up to AN an awning sensation, especially in the mornings of weekdays. But how nice would it be great to know that there is a day ahead of you might be every day just for you? That's what ikigai can do provide you with. It gives you the drive to enjoy life the way you'd like to live it. It's the thrill of enthusiasm. Be a part of your passions everyday and you'll certain be enthralled to keep going with each and every more in the next day and the day that follows. You can enjoy ikigai and you might end up saying "Today was a great day. I was alive today."

Balance, Supervision and Balance

Life regardless of whether you're blessed with ikigai it's not all frozen desserts sparkle, rainbows, and glitter. There are challenges and difficulties, like we all face. We are prone to experience all kinds of loss in expertise and failure, crashing off the proverbial bike and then scalding our knees. The circumstances that we manage toss us curveballs constantly, and can cause us to fall. Everyone has to do the things that they have to do, and not want to do at times. Ikigai will not remove these activities from your daily routine. But, it's at moments that you're looking to make your life's purpose to be the most important. Ikigai will assist in making your decision during difficult times since it helps you achieve the harmony you desire to achieve in your life. Ikigai is the highest amount of an important during times of trouble sadness, sorrow, or pain since it is the reason to be rooked.

Is Ikigai the secret to longevity?

There is a belief that the best aspect about ikigai isn't just happiness. What draws users to this particular form of entertainment is its longevity. It's true that you are able to live longer, close to what we tend to believe. Of Of course, there's no guarantee that you'll make it through Moses or any other person in the same way. However, people from Japan and, especially, Okinawa appear to believe that having a reason to live is essential to live a long and fulfilling life. Being among the countries with the largest populations of centenarians Okinawans are living the proof. It seems that Okinawa might be a 'Blue Zone' which is one of certain places in the world that have above average longevity rates . It also "has one of the largest living female population in the world," as Dan Buettner author of National Geographic shares in his Ted talk, How to live to be 100or more. In fact, when you listen to his talk, you will learn the role of diet and social environment as significant roles in the well-being and health of Okinawans. Okinawans. Dan Buettner additionally goes on to point out that many people are never retired. They are not working due to the fact that they want to, remember, they work due to the fact that they are required to. As a result they are able to keep a vigilance in their body, mind, and soul. Simply speak to associate degrees Okinawan and they will explain that the reason that they have to say goodbye is a result of the fact that they LIVE farewell.

Similar findings are also found in other studies which suggest that ikigai could be connected to longevity:

* Variations in the ikigai of regions (reason(s) to live) in the state of affairs of people. The relationship between the ikigai and family structure the physiological state of affairs and the practical capabilities - Akihiro Hasegawa Ph.D., Toyo Eiwa University

The gray individuals of Japan's foundations and well-being of the participants Social researcher Robert Weiss, Ph.D. Study

* Factors that relate to "Ikigai" in the people who work for an agency of the public for temporary older adults (Silver Human Resources Center) in Japan and gender-related variations Kokoro Shirai, graduate college in Social and Environmental drugs, city University. The study

Is Ikigai spiritual?

Given that Japan is predominantly Shinto and is a part of Buddhism It's a good idea to state that the fundamentals of these two religions are evident in the characteristic of the ikigai. However, the right answers to this question is to take a look at what you consider to be spiritual. If you think that being religious means to adhere to a particular religion one of the others like Buddhism, Shinto, Hinduism, Judaism, Islam, Christianity or a specific religion, then the answer to this question is more like "no" as opposed to "yes."

According to my knowledge, there's anything specific in the Bible regarding ikigai. Or, if there is it could bring you closer to God. But, there is a possibility that if you adhere to the religious teachings and practice brook religion within your life, then going to the midst of your activities. It could fill your life with joy and meaning and help you through tough times and periods of depress. In extraordinary words, dedication toward God or a particular religion maybe your ikigai.

In the end, the concept of religion or the exact doctrine isn't a requirement to adhere to the ikigai. It's religious if you choose to be. So if the purpose of your life is balanced with your religious beliefs that are not secular or spirituality, then absolutely is the answer to the question "Is the ikigai spiritual?" would be a solid, "yes."

Does everyone have Ikigai?

The Japanese consider ikigai exists in all people and is unique to Maine and my beliefs and values that I admire, as it's for you and is a source of joy and direction for your life. It's a private reflection that can be that is reflected through meaning, satisfaction and morals. and joy

Consider your philosophy of thought - what is it?

As with all things in life There are decisions and options, but there aren't correct answers or rules for Igai. There's a wide array of possibilities to travel on and the only guide you have is your own.

Furthermore, the only map you have is the one you draw out prior to you. Plans or goals don't have any other meaning, except keeping you in motion. Ikigai isn't about achieving a specific outcome. It's a continuous process of changing and expanding with you, never ending. Since it's usually the case, it's not the end goal, but more the process. The most important thing is that ikigai is the result you make from it. It may be for some that it could be as extravagant and lavish as working at a center for the elderly or fighting to end the world hunger. For others, it's as delightful and relaxing like planting a garden or making cakes. True ikigai doesn't have any limits, and no boundaries. It's there, regardless of what you want for it to turn out to be. You just need to find your personal philosophy and then live it out. the principles you have chosen to live by.

This is the Demon Within The Room

No matter if you have a vision of your direction and simply beginning out|you'rejust beginning your journey|just starting out} and trying to take your first steps. Although you are in tune with your goal, and like as many people on their journeys, and you could also overcome the biggest obstacle in your path: procrastination. The draw of procrastination is a type of similarity among us all and there are numerous common reasons to procrastinate, such as the fear of failing or lack of motivation being impatient and compulsive. What is affecting people in the American state is totally different from the things that affect you but the final results are similar... You've just have to be proactive to not be faced with the difficulties you want to conquer.

Meet The Challenge Head-On

If you're honest, you'd like to tackle your problems head-on. You'll either be attempting to find for solutions or rush to maintain your pace, or you may put off. There is a risk that a stoppage can end by becoming inactive for each day, followed by two days, and then becoming as per week, and to continue on. If you pause or not taking action you can be assured that your worries towards the motion could ease. By releasing yourself from the task You freed yourself from the fact that you are definitely. But before you can recognize it, you might realize that the lack of harm and then find that you remain in a state of sadness. The worst part is that you'll feel a huge sadness. Procrastination is among the most common and deadly of ailments and the impact it has on the quality of life and happiness is immense. A hockey player. It's often an endless cycle and the worst part is that you can get the desired (albeit negative) outcomes directly and without effort on your part. All the effort and time you have invested would go wasted

Make As Many Steps as You'll Need

Doing nothing is not the way to a full and fulfilling life. If you're feeling a temporary cloud nine, realize that any delay of more than a few days in pursuing your goals is a complete waste of time. There's no other option but to get to get back on the horse and give it a second attempt. The luck of the draw that the great thing with ikigai is that it allows you to only have to go through this repeatedly, and again if you so, choose. Be aware that if be able to get from zero just once then you'll be able to begin again from zero further - at least the moment you're proficient.

How Do You Locate Your Ikigai?

Like the way that life is in flux and consequently, the only constant is the change that happens and what was your dream and passion yesterdaymay not be the same today. The truth is and you will eventually wake up and realize that there is an alternative to the current method. As luck will have it, there is an alternative or more precisely it's possible to find better methods to go about it. Although the experiences of discovery and fulfillment are unique to all individuals, they're also practical actions we can take to aid America. We will look at two popular methods to find your life's purpose, practical and holistic. Each starts by identifying yourself. That is the point at which the path begins.

Chapter 2: Finding Your Way

"The most memorable day of your life is one in which you make the decision that the direction of your life. There are no excuses or excuses. There is no one to trust or to blame. The choice is yours It's an incredible experience and only you are accountable for the quality of it."

Bob Moawad

This chapter we'll look at ways you can determine what you need to be doing when it comes to your job. Sometimes, it's easier to identify what you don't need to know in order to figure out what you need to do.

Are You Confused or In Limbo?

One of the most difficult emotions in the world is being forced to go to work each day realizing that you don't want being there. This can be made even worse when you're stuck and aren't sure what you're doing to the rest of society. It's difficult to know the direction you're headed in and where you'd like to go. It's like you're destined to go "anywhere except there!" The only way to get past this stage is to pinpoint the reason you feel stuck in the place you are. This could be because of various reasons, including fear or uncertainty about the unknown, and what's in store for the future. Change can be scary for the main part, but it's even more so if you're not sure if you're making a right choice.

Sometimes, the stress we feel about our work stems from having to live an ideal career of someone else instead of your own. The best part in life is the fact that you have the ability to succeed in anything you'd like to accomplish by making the best career decisions. Make decisions that align with your values and beliefs. your values system. You'll never be content unless you're living your own goals instead of one that is shared by somebody else. Deciding on your goal is what will push you to a career path that resonates with you and feel like home.'

The Search for the Reason

Finding your 'why' and understanding it is the best way to move away from an environment in which you feel stuck or where you don't feel like you belong. How do you discover your "why"? This, too, requires lots of introspection to get your thoughts feelings, feelings, and even emotions on paper. It's about being able to ask hard questions to discover the reason you're trapped in your present state. One method to accomplish this is creating a mission statement that explains the reason you're in the current job and the reason you've decided to pursue the life you're currently living. This can help you think about your values and what is important to you right now.

As we mature and grow as we gain experience, and get exposed to new concepts, our motives to do things shift. What was significant to us five or even 10 years ago , compared to what's most important today may be totally different. Your circle of friends could be different; or you may be looking to settle down. Here are some tips to help you find your "why," how to find it and what effects it could affect your professional career.

Your "why" shouldn't cause you to feel stressed, overwhelmed or unhappy. It should instead be an integral element in determining what you're looking for on your path to success.

Finding the "why" of what you're supposed to be doing, as opposed to the current situation is among the most difficult challenges to face. It's knowing that you're unhappy with your current situation, and being in a position to pinpoint on what you'd like to do, with evidence-based reasons to support this. Remember that I said at the beginning of the chapter that money isn't always the sole reason to make a move as well as moving might not be the most ideal idea? If you are able to discover the "why" with each of its sub-categories and clearly define each one of them that will give you more clarity on the direction you should follow.

Stephen Warley describes not understanding your "why" as being stuck in "limbo or trapped at the bottom of purgatory." The situation is the same "holding pattern" as the rest of humanity continues to advance and progress. Here is an outline of the suggestions that he gives to define your "why":

The reason you have will guide you to the steps you should undertake in your job.

It can assist you in identifying your purpose in life is.

Once you've figured out the reason behind your decision, your determination and belief to take action will be increased.

* It is your primary drive to achieve your career. It is it is the thing that propels you ahead.

* Your "why" can help define your character as a person, bringing out your personality traits and the qualities that are essential for success.

Your level of productivity will rise since you're doing something you are passionate about.

Your "why" is the basis and the backbone of you "mission assertion" for your professional and for your life.

* It becomes the basis of your work life and weaves a gold thread throughout your career and, in the case of your life.

Finding your 'why' can influence the time, place and how your decisions are taken. A lot of these decisions can affect your future.

* Your "why" will help you develop better understanding of your purpose in life.

Making Career Changes

The choice to change careers isn't always be embraced by everyone. There are times when you'll have to compete with the majority of people. It is possible that you won't be successful right away. It could take some time at first And as all successful people know it is not easy to achieve success. It's always going to require effort and sacrifice. It is possible that you won't see the outcomes for a prolonged duration of time. The people who succeed are typically those who are willing to persevere They're willing to fail when necessary and are accountable for their actions.

When you change your direction and career you might face challenges that you must over come. It's not always easy but they are often necessary to getting to the top.

The process of discovering your "why" starts by identifying and understanding the person you are. This is achieved by utilizing the emotional intelligence aspect of self-awareness. If you believe you have an entire grasp of the person you are and the things you're about, there's actually a amount beyond this. It's about understanding your feelings and emotions and being attentive to the messages they're sending to you at any moment. Self-awareness allows you to communicate with others , by engaging with them at a level that works to benefit both.

If I were to inquire about the actual reason behind remaining at the present time What would you be able to say should you be 100% truthful? Which of the answers below will best explain the reason you're still in your job?

It's a job, and I'm in need of cash.

* I'm in the midst of a massive debt and don't want to be a risk of not having a job.

* My entire circle of friends are employed in this field.

* My spouse is asking me to join this company because of the benefits.

* My parents suggested to me do.

* It's a position I believed was financially viable and had a high potential for earning.

How can you find your "why"?

Do a self-analysis

The suggestions continue to be in line with the self-analysis we started in the first chapter. This requires more thought and writing. This time, I'd like you to write each day about your day's events and things that you've noticed or enjoyed. It could be a matter of events that have occurred at work. Take 15-30 minutes each day to write this information in a notebook that you can refer to it whenever you require.

Keep a journal in the exact same place, take notes of your feelings about any of these:

Principles: What is your moral code of conduct? What is your line between things you're willing to do or not?

What motivates you to reaching your goals? It could be determined by the factors that motivate you.

It is important to examine what you're really committed to? What would you be willing to do in exchange for nothing?

Re-examine your strengths from chapter 1. Are there additional strengths you'd like to add to your initial list? They could be strengths that you're currently using.

What is your ideal day be like? What are you doing? What would be the people you'd consider interacting with or having a conversation with? (This question is very important).

It is essential to keep exact logs regarding your thinking, moods, as well as your actions over a long duration of time in order that you are able to see patterns that are beginning to form.

Examine Your Role

Put your current job under the microscope and examine the situation. Review your career progression step-by-step. What is it that brought you to your current job initially? What are you able to accomplish in the course of your career? Are there any achievements that you are particularly happy about? Did you get any recognition for your achievements? What was the occasion and how did the feeling of being recognized? When do you feel most productive? What time of the day do you feel the most tired? What aspect of your job is the one you are most interested in? This is the area you are able to do easily and makes you feel complete. In each case, look back to your answers and then ask yourself why for each one of them. Be as honestand complete as you can.

Consider the person who inspires you to succeed. Perhaps it's not someone but the reward or reward that inspires you to achieve the things you do. If you have things that make you feel angry or make you angered, note the reasons for these. If you believe that it's something you'll never alter, then you'll need to either accept that fact as it is or choose to change your mind about things that are better.

Do you have any particular things you've been thinking about doing as a kid or activities you love doing during your free time? Two questions arise from this thinking process. The first one is, can you pursue these pursuits during your free time? Second, if you didn't have to worry about finances, would you continue to do what you're doing now?

In the process of identifying strengths and weaknesses which areas do people typically ask your help with?

What service or product would you market and what you could perform in addition to the ones you're currently doing?

What do people in the world require that you have to provide? Can it be used to solve a particular problem or meet the needs of a particular industry or market? If yes, is it an ongoing need? Do you think this will be in the market within the in the next 10 or so years?

Another option is to get those close to you to provide their feedback. You can ask them to provide feedback about what they think your strengths are and what field they think you should be in. However, make certain to ask them reasons for why!

The last few steps to understanding your "why" is to ask the following five questions:

* Are you searching for satisfaction in your job or the ultimate fulfillment at work?

* What can you do to accomplish each day that is simple but still pushes you to grow

as a person and gain more about your work and your personality?

What is it that you are most excited about regarding your current job?

* What is it that gives you the most challenging challenges, yet inspires you in your work?

* What does your ideal job take on?

The Search for Your Ikigai

The term Ikigai is a blend from two Japanese words: iki, which means "life" and kai which means "your motive to exist." Kai can also be seen as the motivation to get up each day. As per People at Heart, it is a combination of hopefulness and doing what you enjoy doing (People at Heart Coach, n.d.).

Your Ikigai is individual to you and are the only one. It gives you the sense of direction and will often guide your in the direction you want to take to be satisfied. It doesn't depend on your identity, the is your job title or how much money you have in your bank or any traditional career-testing strategies. The Ikigai is a native of Okinawa located in Japan and is believed to be from the Heian period of Japanese history (794 until 1185). According to Akihiro Hasegawa, who wrote an article on the topic in 2001. There are a myriad of terms to describe this, however they all are a description of your work experience, when you identify the areas that are overlapping in the Venn diagram (Mitsuhashi 2017).

A study carried out at the end of 2010 by Central Research Services investigated approximately 2000 Japanese males and females on their lives' value based on Ikigai. Just 31% of those interviewed were able to identify work as their Ikigai. It's rarely money that is the primary motivational factor. Although work is an element, it's rarely the sole factor (Suzuki and Central Research Services , Inc., n.d.). As per Yukari Mitsuhashi, "ikigai is the primary reason people get up in the early morning" (Mitsuhashi 2017).

The famous psychotherapist Mieko Kamiya states that "Japanese people believe that the accumulation of little joys and pleasures in everyday life leads to a more satisfying life overall" (Kamiya 1966). The citizens from Japan have the longest-living populations in the world. The average age of women is 87 years old and their male counterparts live around age 81. According to the statistics released provided by the Department of Health, Labor, and Welfare.

Your Ikigai makes you smile through the things that matter for you. It gives you an awareness of your purpose instead of living life according to the rules of others.

Your talents are being utilized for something valuable and you're making an impact in the lives of people whom you meet.

What is the best way to begin to identify your Ikigai?

Two ways you could go about this. Start with an Venn diagram, which has four intersecting circles. Within each of the four circles, note the following:

I'm particularly adept at ...?

* Things I enjoy doing ...?

* What can I get paid for? ...?

* What do we require most? ...?

Another alternative is to create three lists separately:

* Things that you're great at

* What do you want to do

* Your value system

Where these three lists meet is considered to be your Ikigai. It's only after you've put these things into practice that they are your Ikigai (Buettner 2008).).

Other Career Considerations

You've taken your notes on all of these things and have asked yourself these crucial concerns about your next job. Have you thought about all the possibilities? You've identified your interests and the place you'd like to pursue your next profession Are you ready to make the leap?

Kathy Caprino warns of mistakes which are easily made however, they can be avoided if you are aware of the mistakes before they happen. This includes looking at the world from a rose-colored lens. If we're not realistic in our outlook for in the near future, then the most effective method to determine what the future holds is by looking back to the past. Think about what you've accomplished in your career thus far. What's worked and what's gone wrong? There's a reason why you should be honest when answering these questions. You must be accountable, honest and confident about the possibilities that the future will bring. The author identifies five common mistakes that are made by the majority of people looking to change careers.

Not Changing Until Too late

Kathy describes her own experience to illustrate this error. She waited until the situation was such a mess in her former post that she literally fled the position she was so terribly unhappy with. The only thing she was focused on was getting as far from her current situation as far as she could, and she was eventually placed in a job that wasn't the right fit for her. What usually occurs in this situation is it can take more time to figure out your place of origin since you are trying to get rid of all that is even remotely related to the place you've been. This isn't necessarily a good thing since you're wasting your precious time and effort in pursuit of something that isn't right for you. In Kathy's situation she had to put in several more years working on different things before finding the perfect job. She suggests that if there are aspects of your professional life that you'd like to work on, you should start by focusing on them prior to pursuing an entirely new job. It's easier to set your new talents and abilities in a safe security of your current job that pays you and has the security of a steady income, instead of trying to learn these abilities by yourself as you try to establish an entirely new brand or reputation. If there are relationships that require to be repaired, make sure that no matter where you go, there is no chance of repairing the relationships after you've left.

She provides four essential elements to consider when making your next move:

Clarity: Be aware of exactly what it is you're trying to accomplish close enough that you feel as well as taste it.

Engagement: This isn't the time to jump between different options in deciding whether it's worth making the decision to change or not. Once you've committed (like all other obligations) make sure you follow through. If you're not totally in your decision perhaps you shouldn't think about making the move at this point. Be aware that there could be issues that remain unsolved in your current job that have to be resolved first.

Confidence: Being confident in your career choice is what can get you ahead of the pack and allows others to not just admire you, but also to respect you. If you're a softy, or appear apathetic because you're unsure of your abilities, it's the time to think about your plan and if you've made the right choice.

Chapter 3: Four Regions Of The Ikigai

If you've learned about the most fundamental concepts of Japanese philosophy. You will be able see the true significance of Ikigai. Ikigai concept. It is a coherent and unified way of thinking about life that you will now be able to discover the primary purpose of your life. This will help you figure the most important things to you in your life What makes life worthwhile for you personally , and what's worth getting up each day.

There is a belief among the Japanese consider that finding the ikigai to be a first and most vital step to an extended and satisfying life. In general, it is not possible to find it quickly, but it's worth it to begin this thrilling journey into the undiscovered.

It is impossible to predict what could be in store for you at the end which is a reason to have a look at the idea. Therefore, be prepared with plenty of patience as well as the desire to take a take a closer look at your own self - as it is about to begin.

Every masterpiece begins with a blank sheet. Therefore, first grab some paper and a pencil Find a peaceful spot in which you can sit with your thoughts and then let's begin. Place the pen in your hands and create four circles that are interlocking: two on the horizontal plane and 2 on the vertical plan. There must be a central intersection among the four circles. Therefore, larger intersections will also need to be been created between the circles.

The next step is to you must identify your circles, in whatever order you want. Each circle is given any of these words: "What I'm good at", "What I love", "What the world requires" and then "What I might be paid for". Try to assign every one of these four circles of the following phrases. For instance, you could employ nouns and verbs like "parachuting", "surfing", "climbing" etc. They are simple to comprehend and will ensure clarity in the massive amount of information that will soon be created.

This appears to be a relatively straightforward task at first. However, at all times it is best to avoid writing down any terms that pop up in your mind first unless, obviously, you're 100% certain of your answer.

It is best to spend the time to reflect on what activities and items represent the most value to your life, so you can get rid from all superficiality and ultimately be able to get to the heart of the matter. Be attentive to your own thoughts and then look over all four concepts in a circle, one by one.

If you are having trouble or are unsure of the answer, try using the below questions as a reference If you can are able to relate to the things that you excel at The first step is think about whether you've ever prior to being asked by your family or acquaintances about your unique abilities and talents. Did you notice at the school environment that you were praised for any of your personal accomplishments or strengths? Are you of the opinion that there are areas where you could do better than others?

We all know that certifications and references aren't by any way as crucial as real-world experience and skills. However, it's never hurt to reflect on your educational background from time to period: Is the career that you've studied or worked in generally in line with your current abilities? If it isn't, how and where did you learn these skills? Most of the time, individual areas of interest and interests have a lot in common with the skills that can be applied to the individual, particularly since these experience-based experiences usually occurred within engaging in hobbies and other recreational activities. It is also important to think about the issue of your exceptional abilities: Do you believe that you possess these abilities? How can you best apply them to your everyday life to ensure that the world around you can be benefited from these abilities?

The things you cherish may, however differ. Every one of us we have at least a thousand things that make our lives more enjoyable and make our lives much more enjoyable. But that doesn't suggest that these are the only things that have a special space in our souls. It is true that you are a fan of coffee and cakes at lunchtime. Yet it's something that is a part of daily life for a lot of us. Cake and coffee can't be compared to stollen or the Christmas cookie, that you generally only indulge in only once per year. This isn't exclusively about the things you, regardless of the reason you are unable to perform or just indulge in every once in a while. It's more important that these activities inspire you and make your heart move faster (this could cause an emotion). When you are discussing specific things you should think about these questions that will aid you in identifying your own personal Ikigai Do you have the ability to do the activity for long time without feeling tired? Do you remember if you were a fan of this activity as a kid? In this regard others can assist us discover our talents and abilities. But whether these are the things that you are burning for is entirely up to your personal preferences. However, if you've discovered some things that you like then you must consider whether you could imagine doing them for all day. These questions will provide you with a better understanding about the activities you love such as hobbies, interests, etc.

The things you cherish are closely connected to what the world requires in general. Are you sure of what you've got to offer to the world? Or what could the world need from you? Do these things are logical to you? Do you get up each morning contemplating this particular thing or some other thing? Do these activities align to your own personal (or maybe religious) values and are they in line with your personal values that you stand for and actively engage in daily life? What will you leave behind in the world and what will be remembered, and what will the world keep in mind when you're gone? Imagine you vanished without any trace for a long time How long would it take for the world to come to a halt, or what might people around the globe be lacking that the rest of humanity would not be able to emulate as you? What about right now Do you prefer talking to your family and friends about any topic that enthralls you?

If you're unable to answer the question, talk to your closest human beings and ask what their top interests are, or what they believe you would have in the coming years. Be careful not to let yourself be too influenced by opinions of other people or your own thoughts. Don't forget that your image as well as that of others is usually not compatible and that the opinions of others about you won't be 100% to your actual strengths and qualities. However, it is beneficial to get advice from an independent third party , as our families and friends are observant of all the things we do overlook. Also, think about whether there is a certain location where you are desperately needed and people would be missing you so severely if you were to leave? Consider about the contribution you can make to the ongoing or future advancement of our increasingly complicated modern society.

However, ultimately you need to be able to earn money by doing something. Today, it's quite common that later in life, you are not able to do what you imagined as an infant or in relation to your current interests or professional training. If you haven't yet signed a long-term job, you might be thinking about earning your primary income from the job you've studied. Could it be possible to later pursue an occupation in your preferred subject or would you rather pursue your passions and earn a decent living doing them? Both possibilities are open to you, and could be combined in a way that will result in the highest possible profit for you both in terms of financial and personal.

Consider how many of us are dissatisfied with their job Most likely, they were pushed into the wrong direction when they were small children - whether as part of their family, their schools, friends or even their school. Maybe some even been compelled to carry on an ancestral tradition or be part of a artificially constructed system that doesn't necessarily reflect their individual strengths and requirements. The general feeling of discontent with everyday life is usually triggered again and time again as one attempts to escape from the consequences of their actions, or in other words away from reality and the direction of one's life. We all know that life is always in a state of flux or a perpetual state of adjustment.

But, if we deliberately select a position of security or inactivity, our ability to change will slowly diminish as time passes. The ability to adapt keeps us alive in the present and is the basis on which our connection to ourselves and the connection between self and the society at large depend. Certain professional tasks require a significant degree of adaptability, whereas others favor a more passive attitude in every day life. In the end, our lives are shaped by the choices we make every day. This is why crucial choices, like selecting a career, need to be taken with extreme attention. It is also essential to be aware that independence and financial security cannot be achieved one or the other way. If you possess many and diverse strengths and traits they can be utilized effectively in the form of several or more of the activities that you can carry out in your everyday life. By doing this you're making an important contribution to societyand are paid for in a manner that is appropriate. Every person has unique talents that can be used for different functions. If we limit the secret to ourselves in the majority of cases we're missing the true meaning behind this individual talent. Because the world is so that each person is different from the others, even in the smallest way, and so each person is a part of an integrated whole. When we share our abilities and skills to the world, this results in added value that both parties benefit. It is advisable, therefore to think about what people around the globe could benefit from the various aspects of your personality. When you do this you will have nothing to lose. In the event of a disaster you'll only have been through a handful of too numerous experiences.

Did this easy "exercise" gave you the impression that you've gained knowledge about you? It is well-known that it could take some time before you are sure that you've discovered your own Ikigai or the real value of existence. Keep in mind that this occur under stress.

One of the advantages of this approach is in its conceptual ability to adapt: If you decide to perform this task for a number of consecutive days you could get diverse results in each. This is due to the fact that every day is charged emotionally differently. Furthermore, the mood of your individual can have a significant impact on your attitude and you may not get the same mindset following a stressful day, like you would after a quiet day (when you can remain calm and focus only on "essentials").

Do you remember the phrase "Mushoyu-Shin"? Based on this insightful concept of philosophy of The Far East, the heart is a permanent attachment to something, could put people in a downward direction. It doesn't matter if you're experiencing internal struggles with a particular feeling or are dealing with a problem which has been in existence for a long period of time, be careful not to allow your heart to lead to a dead end! Instead, you should try playing the whole game for a longer period of time until you notice the same terms are constantly popping up. Don't focus too much on the material aspects of things. As you've realized, terms such as "matter" or "prosperity" have in a secondary role in Ikigai. Ikigai concept. Therefore, it is best to concentrate on your own interests and values that are within you and everything else is a result of the first.

Eliminate all kinds of negative thoughts and beliefs that can impede you from focusing on your mind and you'll be able to see the true passions you have.

Consider, for instance, something that appears to be straightforward at first glance. If you're a fan of painting more than anything else, but you are unsure of your talents as an artist but this shouldn't stop you from pursuing your talents further. You have discovered only a tiny part that is your individual Ikigai and you are now required to figure out what you can achieve with it. In this instance it is logical to take a painting class first. There is no price without effort is a guarantee that any Japanese will assure you of that.

When we look at the numerous intersections that occur between the various regions of the Ikigai and we will observe that sub-concepts with functional connections arise from this. Let's examine the intersection that has been created between your the personal preferences you have and your unique abilities: This could generally be described as your greatest passion. So, if you've declared that you do not just love playing tennis but you are also extremely skilled at it and have a great deal of experience, you can be certain that it will be more than a hobby for you. In fact, it is an activity worth investing your time and effort into. Personal passions typically are a good source of growth, and can be developed when you have the will, patience and confidence in oneself. They also form one of the main regions of your Ikigai that connects the three other areas of your Ikigai join.

Then, there is the intersection of your passions and what the world requires. The interaction of these two factors will result in your own personal task in your daily life. In the end, if you consider it, everyone is brought into the world with an individual reason for being here: This is evident across the diverse kinds of people who exist. You can find introverts and extroverts artistic and linguistic talents and even cosmopolitan and conservative types. We all have these people in our circle of friends , or at least has similar instances from our own lives. The different kinds of people are all distinguished by distinct qualities and abilities.

This permits the individual to be a part of or even join different social associations that are organized exactly in line with the concept of one's personal traits and interests (for instance, professional sport clubs, trade association or even sports associations).

This is the way society is organized: You may have a memory of the traditional Japanese idea of the person and their role in the society. In Eastern societies, people and their distinct personality are not considered so important as they are in Western societies in which the popular personality cult is the norm. In Japan the social cohesion is an intrinsic value. Therefore, each person is expected to contribute actively to the preservation of the social order as well as take part in the continued growth of it. In this society there is no doubt that it will be insignificant what specific abilities and abilities someone brings to the table since the basic determination serving is the most necessary requirement to be a citizen. Here is the place where the principle of Arugamama is applied and explains how the ability to adapt is utilized in all aspects of daily life. We all recognize that no two people are ever the same, and that everyone has unique talents and abilities. This means that you shouldn't be shocked that certain people are able to do certain things better than others.

Our western culture puts a particular attention to quality and perfection in our daily lives. In Japan it is typical for schoolchildren to, for instance, be taught in all scientific and sports disciplines. Because Japan is not just a robust traditional country but also a well-developed industrial nation. To ensure that the economy is supported optimally and to maintain the high quality of life in society, people are expected to be a type that is an "all-rounder".

But, it doesn't mean that everyone must be an expert in climate-friendly design food, gastronomy, and in the same way fashion-forward. This means you need to be able to adapt to any situation in your life (professional as well as non-professional). No matter if you're a businessman or a basic trader you should be able to comprehend the basics of Japanese poetry, and also be able to dance at least a couple of classic folk songs.

There is no way to be sure of what you can expect the next day or what's going to occur the next day and that's why you need to be ready for anything possible (as as well as for the impossible!). Therefore, it's an overall multi-faceted process which should ensure the capacity to change and consequently the seamless transition of one condition to another or from one state to the next. This is generally a useful strategy to live a normal life since it ensures the continuous flow of energy, and consequently the long-term survival of the person. However, personal mission is more than just a survival plan. Your life's mission is essentially the purpose of your existence. Since what you cherish is what the world wants from you.

Chapter 4: Physical Training To Unlock Your Ikigai

P

Exercises that are hysical and body movements are among the best methods to release your Ikigai. There is a belief that because Ikigai is a product of Okinawa, Japan, which is home to a large number of people who are centenarians, Ikigai holds the key to longevity as well as happiness.

Based on Dan Buettner ('National Geographic' writer), Okinawans above 80 or even 90 are extremely active. Americans who are the same age would rather be at home and read the paper or look at the outside. However, Okinawa seniors are known to walk frequently; they also get awake early and love to singing with their neighbors. They love to tend their gardens prior to or after eating breakfast. They don't perform any intense physical exercises or visit any gym. The key to their longevity is that they never get bored in their day-to-day routines.

I also discovered this secret of longevity through watching my grandparents who were not yet in their 70s and 80s living a full and active life. Today, they like to complete all household chores like cooking and cleaning, washing gardens, grocery shoppingThe list is endless. They're not tech-savvy and don't seem to take any notice. They're too busy living their lives.

If you are in a city, then you might find it difficult to exercise in healthy and natural ways every day. However, you can certainly engage in some physical activities and body movements specific to your body that have proven beneficial for overall health.

It is believed that Eastern exercises that bring your body, mind and mind back into harmony have been practiced for ages.

While these are well-known in the West however, the countries of the east from which they originated have been practicing them to boost health throughout the years.

There is no need to do marathons or go to the gym all day long. All you need to do is add some body activities to your daily routine similar to the Okinawa centenarians.

Practice Eastern exercises frequently is a fantastic way to improve your body's movement. The exercises are well-defined with clear guidelines, which will help to improve flow.

Here are some well-known oriental exercises that are well-known in the eastern world. You can try each one and feel free to select an exercise that will make the body work.

4.1) Radio Taiso

This is a series of exercises using body weight specifically designed to help joints reach their maximum movement. As you go about your daily routine the joint movements usually do not reach fully range, which will eventually cause muscles to shrinkage. The goal of Radio Taiso is to move your entire body through a wide range of motion each day. A regular practice can make you feel more comfortable and continue to improve your performance for longer periods of time.

Radio Taiso exercises can also improve your flexibility and posture, which in turn will help you with basic movements such as sitting on the floor or rising from the chair. Additionally, these easy exercises, when performed in the morning, could assist in increasing the flow of blood throughout your body. This can aid in reducing stiffness that has built up as well as loosen joints and help to energize your whole body.

Prior to the Second World War, instructions for the Radio Taiso exercises were transmitted through radio. This is why the word "Radio was added to the name. However, Japanese people of today usually practice these moves by watching videos of the movements via the web or on a TV channel.

Inspiring a sense of harmony among people is the main motive behind conducting Radio Taiso exercises. They are usually done in groups, generally during school before the start of classes. They can also be performed in offices prior to starting the day.

If Radio Taiso activities are done in groups, it's usually in a large hall for reception or on a field for sports and typically involves the use of an audio system. It will take about 5 or 10 minutes to complete the exercises, based on whether you perform specific exercise routines or do them all. The exercise focuses on strengthening joint mobility and dynamic stretching.

The most well-known Radio Taiso exercise involves lifting both arms above your head, then, in a circular motion moving your arms downwards. It's the perfect method to get your body moving and energized. body. It's also an simple mobility exercise that is focused on moving the most joints possible.

This workout may seem simple in your mind, however, in the type of lifestyle that individuals lead nowadays, they often spend their days not raising their arms above their heads. If you consider your daily routine, you'll realize how long your arms are slack when using phones or computers. Or reading books.

The only occasion you raise your hand above the head level is when reaching for something that is on top of the cupboard or closet. Radio Taiso exercises will allow you to learn the fundamental body moves.

There are a variety of Radio Taiso exercises videos available on the internet. You can learn Radio Taiso while watching these videos.

4.2) Yoga

It is a body-mind practice founded on the ancient Indian philosophical principles that date back to 5,000 years. Yoga is becoming extremely popular among millennials in recent times because it aids in gaining control over your body and mind , and improve your overall health.

There are many yoga styles that incorporate breathing techniques, meditation as well as physical postures and relaxation. Yoga practices help build the foundation to develop healthy habits, such as self-control as well as non-attachment and self-inquiry.

The practice of yoga is an avenue that allows you to make conscious choices to live a balanced and happy life. The word yoga comes from the word 'yuj' which is a sign of improved internal state like peace, happiness, or clarity.

In today's world we are in a unique position to be connected with yoga via a wide variety of channels. It is possible to practice yoga in a variety of methods ranging from gyms to schools, studios or community centers, as well as other outdoor spaces to social media platforms and online videos that allow you to completely be immersed in. It is also possible to attend conferences, training sessions and retreats throughout the globe.

There are many ways to practice yoga that place you in the best place to begin or increase your practice. It is possible to modify the practice according to your body's needs and health.

4.2.1) The benefits of Yoga

Yoga can improve your flexibility and strength. Yoga movements can be done by anyone. Yoga is not only for people who wish to be in a state of meditation or feel their toes. Some yoga routines are intended to relax, while in others, you'll require more movement. The majority of yoga styles are based on asanas that concentrate on learning postures that require attention and breathing.

* Increases flexibility Yoga exercises aid in stretching muscles and improve mobility. You'll feel less tired or stiff. As you continue to practice you'll begin to notice the benefits of flexibility. Numerous

studies have shown that yoga instructors generally increase their flexibility after just eight weeks of yoga , by up to 35 percent.

* Increase Strength Certain styles of yoga like Ashtanga and power yoga are extremely physical. You can build your strength and endurance by practicing these styles of yoga. Certain yoga styles like Hatha or Iyengar are not as vigorous. These yoga styles may assist you in attaining the benefits of endurance and strength. Certain yoga postures like the plank, the upward dog and downward dog will aid in building strength for your upper body. Certain standing postures help to build the strength of your quadriceps, abs, and hamstrings. This is especially true when you are able to hold these postures for longer durations of breath. Yoga postures such as the chair pose as well as upward dog can aid in strengthening ones lower back. If you practice these postures

correctly, they are able to help strengthen the abdominal muscles the strength and endurance.

* Improves Posture: If your muscles are stronger and flexible this automatically improves your posture. The majority of sitting and standing postures aid in strengthening your core muscles since the muscles in your core are needed to hold and support every pose. A strong core can aid you to sit (with straight backs) as well as stand up tall. Yoga can help increase awareness of your body. If you're slumping or slouching you'll be able to notice it quicker and be able to modify your posture.

* Improves Breathing. Practicing yoga usually involves the practice of focusing on breathing. This helps to relax your body and mind. Certain styles of yoga also require exact breathing techniques. Be aware that yoga isn't as aerobic as cycling

or running. Only certain types of yoga are as vigorous.

* Relieve stress: Yoga may lower stress levels and help you feel calmer and more peaceful. Certain styles of yoga utilize meditation techniques that help to calm your mind. While practicing yoga, paying attention to your breathing can help lessen stress.

* Heart-friendly: Engaging in yoga can reduce the heart rate as well as reduce blood pressure. Yoga is also a great way to reduce cholesterol and triglyceride levels and enhance the function in your body's immune system. Patients suffering from heart disease, high blood pressure or who suffered from strokes will definitely benefit from yoga.

4.2.2) Yoga Types

Modern yoga is centered around exercise breath techniques along with flexibility, as well as overall strength. Yoga is also a great way to enhance physical and mental well-being.

There are a variety of yoga styles, but there is no particular style is effective or true to different styles. For maximum benefit you will need to pick the style that is appropriate for the fitness levels of your.

The following are the various yoga styles and varieties:

* Ashtanga yoga The Ashtanga yoga style utilizes the ancient yoga philosophies and concentrates on executing six well-known poses that connect every move to the breath. This type of yoga became very popular during the 70s.

"Hatha Yoga": In the general sense any style of yoga that involves physical poses is known as the hatha yoga. The style of yoga typically serves for a brief introduction into the basics in yoga poses.

* Bikram yoga: Bikram or "hot" yoga is generally performed in heated rooms that can reach temperatures of 100 degrees and humidity of 40 percent. The style of yoga consists of two breathing exercises and 26 postures.

* Jivamukti yoga: The word Jivamukti means 'liberation while living. This type of yoga incorporates spiritual practices and instructions that do not focus on the postures but rather on the swift movement between poses. This type of focus is called vinyasa. Every yoga class examines a specific topic through singing, meditation yoga scriptures asana, music and pranayama. The yoga practice can be physically demanding.

* Iyengar yoga This style of yoga focuses on getting the right alignment for each pose using the use of various props, such as blocks, blankets and chairs, bolsters, and straps.

* Kundalini yoga: The word kundalini refers to a 'coiled-shape that resembles snake. This style of yoga is a method of meditation that aims to let go of the trapped energy. The practice usually begins by chanting and then ends by singing. Between these, the practice includes pranayama, meditation, and asanas that are designed to give an exact result.

* Kripalu yoga The Kripalu yoga style gives its students everything they need to learn, understand and accept their bodies. As an instructor, you'll be able to determine your own personal level of practice by observing and learning from your body. The sessions usually begin with gentle stretching and breathing exercises. They are followed by a series of postures and a final meditation.

* Power Yoga: Yoga enthusiasts created this active and athletic yoga style in the

latter half of the eighties. It is an adaptation of traditional Ashtanga yoga.

* Viniyoga: The style of yoga is a great fit for anyone regardless of physical abilities. Viniyoga students undergo intensive training to become expert in the anatomy of yoga as well as.

* Sivananda: Based on a five-point approach This yoga style is focused on breathing, relaxation and fitness, positive thinking and eating habits. Five elements are incorporated to help you live a healthier yogic life style. Sivananda yoga is typically comprised of the 12 basic asanas, which include sun salutations and savasana.

Prenatal Yoga: The style of yoga is characterized by postures specifically made for women expecting. Prenatal yoga not only aid in maintaining women's health throughout pregnancy, but also assist to get them back in form post-pregnancy.

*Yin: Also known by the name of Taoist practice, the Taoist style is a tranquil and meditative method of practice. This style of yoga helps relieve tension in a variety of crucial joints like the ankles, knees and knees as well as the whole back, hips shoulders, neck, and back. Yoga is a form of passive posture that is to say, the majority of the work and force is borne by gravity.

The * restorative style of yoga includes relaxation techniques. When you are in a class of restorative yoga it is performed by performing the basic poses of 4 or 5 with props like bolsters and blankets to get into a deep relaxed state. There is no need to make an effort to maintain the posture.

4.3) Tai Chi

Also known as meditation-in-motion, Tai Chi is one of the best ways to ease stress. Though it was originally developed for self-defense purposes, Tai Chi has evolved into a graceful method of slow-body moving exercise. It is now used to treat various health issues that include stress reduction.

Tai Chi helps promote calmness by using fluid, gentle movement of the body performed in a tranquil and focused way, accompanied by deep breathing. It's a self-paced method of gentle stretching and physical exercises. Every Tai Chi posture smoothly flows from one to the next without stopping, and the continual movement of your body.

There are many distinct Tai Chi styles, and each style can highlight the various Tai Chi techniques and principles. Within every Tai Chi style, there are many variations. Certain styles might concentrate on general health, while other styles might focus on the self-defense component that is a part of Tai Chi.

Tai Chi is considered safe for people of all fitness levels and ages, as it exerts only a small amount of strain and impact on your muscles and joints. Because it's a low-impact workout it is especially beneficial for those who might not be able to exercise normally.

Because Tai Chi is inexpensive and requires no equipment or special tools It is attractive. It is possible to practice it at any time in the indoors or outdoors, and as a couple or in solitude. But pregnant women and those with joint pain such as back pain, fractures and hernias or severe osteoporosis should consult their doctors prior to practicing Tai Chi. A few modifications or avoidance of certain poses may be suggested to them.

4.3.1.) Advantages to Tai Chi

When you master Tai Chi correctly and perform it consistently, it will assist in developing a positive mindset to improve the overall quality of your health as well as wellbeing. The following are the most well-known advantages that can be derived from Tai Chi:

* Happier mood

* Lower depression, stress and anxiety levels

* Increased stamina and endurance

* Increased capacity to run

* Increased muscle strength

* Greater balance, agility and flexibility

* Immune system improvement

* Better sleep quality

* Reduction in blood pressure

* Improvement in the symptoms of congestive failure

* Less joint pains

* Reduced risk of falling among older adults.

Enhanced general well-being

To master Tai Chi, you must get help from a certified Tai Chi teacher to learn the proper techniques and enjoy the maximum benefits. You can purchase DVDs or rent eBooks to study Tai Chi on your own.

A Tai Chi trainer doesn't need to be certified or possess any specific training program certification. You can inquire about their experiences and their training and, if you can ask for suggestions.

The Tai Chi trainer can teach you breathing techniques as well as specific positions. Trainers can also instruct you in practicing

Tai Chi safely, particularly when you suffer from chronic illnesses or injuries, coordination or balance issues. If you do not follow your Tai Chi techniques properly, you could be injured.

Tai Chi doesn't come with any adverse consequences. When you've mastered Tai Chi, you'll gradually become more comfortable doing Tai Chi on your own. You may also want to think about groups of Tai Chi sessions if you enjoy being around other people.

Certain Tai Chi benefits may last for 12-weeks or more. If you keep practicing Tai Chi for a longer periodof time, you'll be able to enjoy higher benefits and be able to master the art.

In order to establish a routine engaging in Tai Chi every day at the same time and in the same spot could be beneficial. If you have a schedule that isn't consistent it is possible to practice Tai Chi wherever you are for a couple of minutes. When you are in stressful situations, like for example, a stressful meeting at work or a road block, you could do the calming Tai Chi mind-body exercises without doing any movements with your body.

4.4) Qigong

Pronounced chee-gung It's the research and practice of nurturing vital life force using a variety of methods, including breathing techniques, postures guided imagery and meditation.

Qi is a reference to air or breath and is considered to be the life force. The people who practice it believe that this vital force is able to penetrate and be a part of everything. Qi is related to the Sanskrit term 'prana' the Greek word 'pneuma as well as the Western medical concept of 'bioelectricity.'

Gong means "effort" or "work," and also refers to the effort you put into any activity or skill that takes time, patience and repetition to reach perfect. Through practice and learning one strives to increase their ability to alter Qi in order to reduce illness, boost self-healing and increase longevity.

4.4.1) Exercise Qigong

The following are two kinds of Qigong techniques:

* External Elixir (Wai Dan): This involves physical and mental concentration as well as moves.

Internal Elixir (Nei Dan) It involves visualisation or guided imagery as well as the practice of sitting meditation.

In accordance with Qigong traditional instruction, newcomers begin by learning the physical movements that are in sync and breathing methods. They do various exercises that are that are similar to Tai Chi to perfect each move or posture. After mastering the fundamental moves and postures then the second step will be to master moving meditation, which is to understand the fluctuation in energy flow, or the subtle movement of it that occurs within the postures, movements as well as transitions and breathing patterns.

Qigong is a series of poses that remain in place for long periods of time. These positions are like yoga postures and fall in the category of meditation that is still. These Qigong poses can aid in increasing energy flow and build up your legs. Certain Qigong exercises include the practice of sitting and meditation, which focuses on gaining a better understanding of your body, mind, and breathing.

You can do sitting, moving, or still meditations, with or without visualisation.

Visualization enhances the intensity of your practice because it allows you to direct the flow of energy according to the visualization you have.

Chapter 5: Antiaging Secrets

Small things that add up to an enjoyable and long-lasting life

Since the beginning of time and a half, we've managed to add 0.3 years each year to our life duration. But what if we could have the technology to increase a year in the life expectancy of each year? It is possible that we would achieve biological longevity after having reached the "escape speed" of ageing. The Escape Velocity of Aging and the Rabbit Think of a sign that is far from the present with numbers on it that represents the age at the time of your death. You get closer to the sign each year you remain. After hitting the button you are dead.

Imagine a bunny walking with the sign and heading toward the sign. Every year, the rabbit could be just half an hour. The rabbit will come at you in the middle, and end up dying.

But what happens do you think if the rabbit walks through your life in the span that is one-year? You wouldn't be able to catch the rabbit, and you also would never pass away.

The innovation is the speed at which a rabbit can run towards the future. The faster we can make the rabbit run, the faster we can advance knowledge and science inside our own bodies.

The speed of escape for aging is when the rabbit can run at or above a pace of one year per year, and we are invincible.

Scientists who are looking towards the future, believe that within the next few decades , we will be able to achieve this speed of escape. A lot of scientists are less optimistic in their predictions that we'll reach a point where we won't be able of achieving an age limit regardless of how much technology we have. For instance, biologists believe that after 120 years, cells cease to regenerate.

A youthful mind, an active body The adage "mens Sana corpore Sano" ("a well-balanced mind within a sound body") includes a great deal of wisdom. It teaches that body and mind are essential and that each is a direct result of the other. Maintaining a healthy, flexible mind has been proven to be among the primary factors that keep us youthful.

Being young in mind typically helps you live an active lifestyle that slows the process of getting older.

A lack of physical activity can have negative consequences for our bodies and emotions, a lack of mental exercise can be harmful for us because it causes our synaptic connections and nerves to become weaker, which eventually hinders our ability to adapt to the environment around us.

This is why getting your brain working is essential.

There's a difference between what someone's right is and what they wish to do. This is because individuals, particularly the older, are more inclined to do things the same way they've always done their lives. The issue is that once the brain develops patterns that last for a lifetime, it is no longer required to think. When it is on autopilot the tasks can be completed quickly and efficiently, and sometimes in a way that is beneficial. It creates a tendency to stick to routines and trying to challenge the brain with new knowledge is the most effective way to shake them.

When presented with new information that stimulates the brain, it also revitalizes the existing connections. This is why exposing your mind to new ideas is essential, even if moving outside of your comfort zone can cause somewhat anxious.

The effects of behavioral training have been proven in a clinical study. The first time you begin exercising your brain through any task, "he says. "So it's a bit complex at first, however the training is still in place because you are able to accomplish it. You'll recall the second time it's simpler to master, not harder as you get faster at this. This has a profound impact on the way an individual. It's a change of its own that can affect not only the results obtained, but also the self-image of the person. "This definition of"visual exercise" visually-based exercise "may appear a bit formal, however, simply being with other peopleby playing games for instance, provides new stimulation and can help to avoid the loneliness that can be a result of solitude.

Cells are beginning to grow when we're at the end of our 20's. However, this process is affected by mental energy and interest as well as an interest in learning. Making new discoveries and observing something new every day or playing games, and engaging with other people are essential anti-aging strategies that benefit the mind. In reality, positive thinking in this regard can provide better mental health benefits.

Stress: Convicted of killing the longevity

Many people are feeling older than they actually are. Research into the causes of premature aging have revealed that stress has a lot contribute to it. Additionally, in times of stress, the body's breakdown occurs more quickly. In the American Institute of Stress studied the degenerative process and discovered that depression can be the cause of many of the health issues.

Researchers at Heidelberg's University Hospital in Heidelberg performed an experiment that involved exposing the young doctor to a job interview. They made the task even more difficult by forcing him to complete 30 minutes of complex maths questions. Then, they took one drop of blood. They found that antibodies react to stress in the same way that they respond to viruses, by releasing proteins that trigger the immune system to respond. It is important to note that this response not only neutralizes the infectious agent, but can also destroy healthy cells which causes premature ageing.

The research was carried out at an institution called the University of California, taking the evidence and measurements of thirty-nine people with elevated stress levels due to one of their children's diseases as well as comparing them to measures taken from those with healthy children and low stress levels. The results show that stress triggers the cell to age by degrading structures, such as telomeres that trigger cell regeneration and the aging in our cell. The more painful the stress is the more cell's degenerative effects, as evidenced by research.

How does he handle stress?

The workforce is at a rapid pace nowadays, and are constantly in a battle. Stress is a physiological response in this heightened state of awareness that the body perceives the information as potentially dangerous or threatening.

This is a good reaction, in the ideal scenario, since it allows us to survive in dangerous situations. This strategy has been used during our development to face the harsh conditions and to avoid the predators.

Pituitary gland stimulation producing hormones that release corticotropin. Corticotropin then circulates throughout the body via the sympathetic nervous system through the alarms that go off in the brain. Cortisol and adrenaline activation is then triggered in the adrenal gland. Adrenaline improves the rate of breathing and heart rate, and also helps us train our muscles for a workout and enables the body to react to any danger. Cortisol increases your body to produce dopamine as well as blood glucose. Blood glucose is the reason we are "strong" and allows us overcome obstacles.

Modern humans operate all the time, and are always alert to the possibility of a risk.

Are available 24 hours a days on the internet in search of updates on the mobiles of their phones.

The brain associates to a predator's danger the touch of a phone or an e-mail.

Cortisol levels that are elevated circulate throughout the body on a constant basis and can cause many health problems that include adrenal exhaustion as well as chronic fatigue syndrome.

Cave Dwellers Most of the time felt tension was lessened in the most limited of situations.

The warnings were true that at any moment, the perpetrator could lose his life.

The low doses of cortisol and adrenaline helped keep the body in a safe place during the time of danger.

They are beneficial when used in moderation. They help us overcome issues that arise in our lives. However, the stress that people are exposed to is evidently negative.

The effects of stress over time can have an effect that is degenerative. An extended state of emergency impacts the memory-related brain cells and can delay in the production of hormones, the absence of which can cause depression. The side effects of this include sleeplessness, irritability, anxiety, and elevated blood pressure.

Therefore, while challenges can be beneficial for keeping our minds and body in good shape We must alter our stressful lifestyles to avoid our bodies from ageing prematurely.

If the threats we encounter are real or not, stress can be a evidently a disorder that causes anxiety, but is also psychosomatic. It affects every aspect of our digestion to body.

It's the reason that avoiding stress is crucial in reducing the impact that stress causes and the reason why a number of experts suggest that we take note of.

The principle behind this method of reducing stress is to examine the self: to observe the responses we make regardless of the influence they have received from practices, in order to be aware of these. We are able to communicate with the here and now while reducing thoughts and thoughts that appear to be spinning beyond control.

"We must try to stop the autopilot within an endless circle that is driving us. We have also met people who eat their meals on the phone or on the television while talking. When you ask them if their breakfast they had just eaten has onions in it, but they are unable to answer. The best way to attain an enlightened state is to practice meditation. This assists in removing the information from the outside world that influences us. It is possible to achieve this through yoga, breathing exercises and body scans as well.

To master knowledge, it takes a lengthy process of training However, with a little amount of practice, we can be taught to concentrate our minds. This reduces depression and helps us live longer.

A bit of stress can be good for you , however continuous, extreme stress is an acknowledged challenge, both mentally and physical health has been proved to be beneficial when stress levels are low.

Over the course of more than 20 years of studying a variety of research areas, it was found that people who had an unrelenting level of stress was able to overcome obstacles and put their hearts and souls into their work to achieve excellence and live longer than those who opted for an easier lifestyle and retired earlier. The researcher concluded that a moderate dose of stress is a great thing because those with less stress adopt better lifestyles, are less smokers and drink less alcohol.

Given this, it's no wonder that many of the supercentenarians-people who live to be 110 or more-who we'll encounter in this book talk about having led busy lives and worked long into old age.

The majority of sitting can cause you to age.

In particular, specifically in particular in the Western globe, an rise of sedentary behavior has resulted in a variety of illnesses like obesity and hypertension that in turn impact the longevity of people.

Being too active at work or at home, not only reduces lung and body capacity, but it also increases appetite levels and decreases the desire to take part. Being inactive can cause weight gain, imbalances in diet and cardiovascular diseases osteoporosis, as well as certain types of cancers. Recent research has shown that there is a link between a lack of physical exercise and the degrading of telomeres over time in the immune system. This alters certain cells, and, consequently the entire organism.

It's a concern throughout the life span and not only for adults. The children of the obese are afflicted with an excessive amount of weight as well as the associated risks and health issues and that's why adopting an active and healthy lifestyle from an early age is vital.

Being less sedentary is easy and requires only some effort and a few adjustments to your daily routine. You can live a more active lifestyle that helps us feel better both inside and outside-we simply need to incorporate the following to our daily routines such as:* Walk to work, or simply do a little exercise for at minimum twenty minutes each day.

Instead of using an elevator or escalator utilize the foot. This is ideal for as well, your joints, breathing as well as your breathing system.

Participate in fun or social activities to avoid spending all of your time watching television.

• Replace the fruit with a fast food, and you'll get less temptation to snack, and more nutrition within your food.

* Get plenty of sleep. It's best to sleep between seven and nine hours but not more than that makes people feeling tired.

* Join a youth group dogs, other dogs, or join a team of athletes. This not only

improves the physical body, it also helps to strengthen the mind and improves self-esteem.

Be aware of your day-to-day life to recognize and replace negative habits with more productive ones.

We'll help regenerate our minds and bodies through these incremental changes, and increasing our lives expectancy.

The most sought-after secret of models

As we age physically and mentally, both physically and mentally one of the aspects that can tell us more about aging of people is their skin. It can take on different hues and shapes based on the changes that take place under the skin's surface. Most people who earn an income as models are known to stay up late in the night prior to an event, between 9-10 hours. This results in a firm skin, smooth face, as well as a healthy glowing shine.

Research has proven that sleep is an important anti-aging mechanism in that we create the hormone melatonin when we sleep, a hormone which exists naturally in our bodies. Due to our diurnal as well as nighttime patterns the pineal gland creates it by releasing serotonin, the neurotransmitter in our brains. It is involved in our sleeping and waking cycles.

Melatonin is a potent antioxidant can help people live longer. It also has the following advantages:

1. It boosts the immune system.

2. It has the cancer-protecting component.

3. It aids in the production of natural insulin.

4. Slows the progression of Alzheimer's disease.

5. Reduces the risk of osteoporosis, and also helps prevent heart failure.

Melatonin is an excellent help in maintaining youthfulness, due to all of these reasons. But it is important to remember that the growth of melatonin decreases after the age of 30. It is countered by eating healthy food to gain more calcium.

* To absorb enough sun each day.

* Make sure you have enough time.

Avoiding alcohol, heat cigarettes, heat and caffeine, which all make it harder to have a restful night's sleep and rob us of the melatonin that we require.

Scientists are trying to determine if artificially increasing the production of melatonin will prolong the aging process. It would confirm the notion that within us, we have the key to immortality.

Anti-aging Perceptions

Brain has an enormous influence on the body's health and speed at which it gets older. The majority of doctors believe that the secret to keep your body in good health is to keep your mind active-- which is a key aspect of ikigai - and not allow ourselves to be defeated when faced with the challenges of our lives.

One study, conducted in Yeshiva University, showed that people who live the longest are those who have two traits that are common to all people that include a positive attitude and a high level of emotional awareness. That is, the people who are currently on the path towards success are able to face challenges with a positive attitude and are able to manage their emotions.

Being in a state of loss or feeling stoic, a positive attitude may aid in keeping your youth, as it decreases levels of anxiety and depression as well as stabilizes behavior. This can be observed by living a relaxed, purposeful life as well as the higher lifespan of other society.

Many supercentenarians and centenarians shared similar characteristics: they led hectic lives, which were usually difficult, yet they knew how to manage these difficulties with a positive outlook and not be overwhelmed by the challenges they faced.

Alexander Imich, who became the oldest living person around the globe at 111 in the year 2014, recognized that he was blessed with genes, but also acknowledged that other aspects are also contributing: "Life that you lead is even more crucial for your survival"

An ode to long-term health

In the course of our visit to Ogimi which holds record-breaking Guinness record for longest-lived people, a woman who was about to reach 100 sang this song to us. It was a mixture from Japanese along with local dialect: to be secure and live an extended life take a tiny amount of anything and have fun. sleep in early, wake up early and go out for a walk.

We enjoy peace each day, and we enjoy the journey.

We're getting along well with our friends to live a long and happy life. an extended life.

Autumn, spring, as well as winter. We enjoy the different seasons with laughter and fun.

The trick is to not be irritated by how old your fingers appear to be. from the feet up to the top of your head.

If you don't stop working to improve your vision, the age of 100 will be upon you. How to become old and still be alive In Okinawa Island in Japan, most 100-year-olds reside among 100,000 people.

Here's how to Keep Your Life Alive and Never Get Older.

Reduce stress in a conscious way anxiety: Stress has a negative impact to our wellbeing. The authors offer a few suggestions regarding how you can manage stress better. Meditation is a form of stress management , but it also helps you remain focused even in the midst of everyday tasks.

Keep active physically Writers explain their belief that the "enemy of being young" is sitting. We offer a few ways to get around every day. Take a walk or work out for at least 20 minutes each day. Have amusement. Make sure you don't use elevators or escalators, or elevators, just your legs. According to the authors: Rotating your body in a relatively intense manner can lead to more longevity.

It is crucial to get enough rest and to sleep.

Food: Naturally, a healthy diet is vital. The Okinawa diet is often referred to"wonderdiet. "wonderdiet" For starters having a wide diverse diet and not overeating is crucial. The centenarians eat only food. There are times when they pick only once each week and then use sugar. They consume a lot of sweet potatoes and tofu as well as about 300 grams of veggies every day. They consume a wide range of food items, and are mostly based on vegetables. They also consume carbs daily and consume tiny portions of everything frequently throughout the day.

* It is essential to create close social bonds with your family, friends or neighbors. Moai groups were established on Okinawa to create the concept of a social network. The older members of these communities are often sharing their experiences in difficult times, and also helping each other.

Maintain your mental strength It is crucial to be able to use your brain. This is possible through stimulation of the brain or searching for new situations.

* Take a walk in the nature, enjoy yourself and smile.

Chapter 6: What's Your Igai?

There's a method to interpret your ikigai. It is based on the traditional Japanese tradition from which the concept was first conceived. It is built around four questions which must be addressed to a specific question.

It is possible to make your Venn scheme by drawing the converging circles in the ikigai picture and find your responses to the fundamental questions in the massive outer circles. This lets you quickly determine which words are present in the contiguous and reverse areas of your graph.

What do you like about it?

This research is aimed at understanding what you find amusing, fascinating and convincing

What are you able to do on your own so that you don't need to draw attention to the financial value of creation?

How can you put your energy into a lengthy trip or a weekend?

What stimulates you and helps you feel more energetic when you're doing it?

What can you debate vigorously for a time?

What the world really needs?

This study aims to clarify what it could bring in the world through its style of living, or even its family.

What issues in your general public could you assist you in understanding right away?

What issues in your community/everyone affects you personally?

Do people want to let their possessions behind to purchase your products?

Does your work have any impact 10 years (or even one hundred years) from now?

How do you make yourself acceptable?

This research seeks to give the significance of his distinctive advantages such as his talents and gifts.

What areas of your current job do you think it is readily acceptable?

What do you do to be among the top employees in your workplace environment or network (or even globally)?

If you had a bit more training and experience, you could you become one of the best in your field?

What You Can Be Paid

The question is about things you could put on your table, regardless of whether it's something that you enjoy or you don't.

Have you recently been compensated for the work you do? Have you ever been compensated for your work? If not, have the other workers paid for this work?

Are you sure that in the future you'll be doing exactly what you are doing? Are you sure that you will be able to make a living working this way?

Spend a few minutes to think of sentences, expressions and ideas that pop up for you within each circle. Then, you can decide how much to search for common cover areas. If you know the answers to these questions, begin to look at the various areas where they intersect.

Each of these parts as well as the connections they have with one another. The aim is to have all of the parts that cross in harmony, right at the center location of the map. This is the way to achieve your ikigai. It is the key to a successful, happy and long-lived life.

The most important thing to live an extended and happy life is to have the same purpose. The first step in living in a way that's designed is to take back control of his life and Japanese Igai's ideas are an excellent tool to achieve it. It may take many years or even years to discover the reason in the first place. However, show moderation; you deserve it.

Be sure to take care of her in everything she has as quickly as possible. Finding your ikigai can be an extremely enriching process and it's worth the effort and time it requires.

It's interesting to note that only 25% of the concept is actually about work. In the Japanese review just 31 percent of people thought their job was their ikigai. Examine this from a nation that is known for addiction to work, there were the majority of Americans who claimed in the Pew Research Center study that their personality was influenced by their work.

That's why I didn't know why I was not happy with my high-life; I was constantly looking at the outcomes, and then trying to figure out the next. But, although writing books is something to be proud of, Garcia says, it isn't an ikigai. "It's an aim. "Ikigai En; I have to write down and become required to do so in order that my thoughts will change the world. "Mixing my acceptance and lovingly communicating - with the world's needs , and being paid for it takes the helm and back between the center.

But, you don't get up in the morning with ikigai. The term "natural" refers to the ability to find it with efficiency. To discover yours, you must ask these questions.

How often do you feel At Peace?

Take a look at the moments where you feel more at ease or "in in the moment. "For the person who is in this state, it is possible to cultivate or by singing or taking part in basic political activities. It may be connected to your job or not at all is it said Chloe Carmichael, Ph.D. She is a New York therapist in private practice.

"In the event that you're seeking some reason to be in your job, you must to know the reason which explains the motive," he says. "Is it appropriate to say that your job is to transmit, educate or inspire others to create an item that enhances the lives of people? On the other side, can your work create a greater impact on your fellow citizens like, for instance, providing a house or property, strength, or your family? What is your answer?

It could also be a cause of Igai".

What are their qualities?

Take a look at what you take note of what you like and. It's often shockingly simple to get to the root of what creates the most difference, according to life coach Cortney McDermott. She is the one who created transformation that starts within your own mind. One suggestion: write down the names of the four people you are extremely respectful of This could be your mom or Opah and then write five characteristics for each.

"The traits you observe like consideration and tolerance, or a positive attitude are likely to be the traits you desire within your own life," McDermott says. These qualities should determine your actions and reasoning. When you have achieved these conditions, by being at peace as you prepare a fresh person for work and work, you will be able to approach your ikigai.

Do you see the drawings?

For many Igai isn't fixed, but it does grow and evolves throughout the years, Garcia says. "Some might discover it that they have young children. As youngsters grow older and mature, they must change their energy. What is more stable are repetitive arguments, or things that are often abandoned and make you happy." They may need your ikigai.

Danielle Dineen, 34, has had a great career, but she's been a victim by her work. She realized that her most enjoyable moments were outside of work, usually during gatherings with friends who could talk about their struggles to her. "I enjoyed listening to people and was able to persuade them to be open and discover ways to be happier or to find better solutions. This helped her remember Central School as well as high school, when she was the source of suggestions to her classmates."

This led Dineen to become an expert for social services. In his current role as an expert, he applies his compassion and listening abilities (the circles "what you're acceptable to do" as well as "what you cherish" floating) in his job (the circulars "what the world requires" and "what will you get for it"). Explosion: "ikigai."

Chapter 7: The Venn Diagram With The Purpose

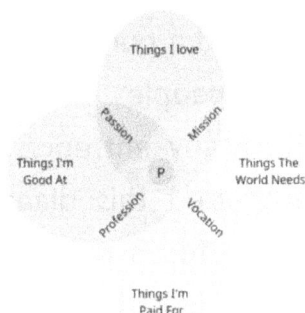

The Purpose Venn Diagram is a symbol of the path that we can be following to discover the meaning to our existence. It was invented by Andres Zuzunaga who was an author and astrologer. The diagram has been misunderstood by those who believe it's Ikigai. It is not. Purpose Venn Diagram does not represent Ikigai since Ikigai is a very old philosophical system that originated in Japan. But, the Purpose Venn Diagram can be a method of finding

Ikigai that is extremely thorough and comprehensive. It's never a bad idea to search for Ikigai using these methods and directions.

Zuzunaga developed a purpose diagram in order to help people discover their purpose in life. Many entrepreneurs and coaches have utilized this diagram as a way to help them focus their minds and focus their lives. This is, basically the way to identify your Ikigai. Its Purpose Venn Diagram appears like this:

The four principal ellipses are the lists you're required to complete in order to determine your purpose. Between these ellipses, it is possible to uncover certain aspects in your lives. There is your passion, your mission as well as your profession and your vocation. The "P" in the middle is a sign of the purpose behind it. Zuzunaga suggests that you find your purpose by doing things that bring you happiness, those you excel at, the ones could be transformed into a career and, lastly giving you purpose because the world is in need of them. There are many parallels between Zuzunaga's search to find a goal and Ikigai. These similarities are significant and the diagram is extremely useful in determining the meaning and significance in our lives that it's become an equivalent in the west to that Japanese notion of Ikigai. The diagram is drawn using the term "Ikigai" in the middle instead of P for reason which was the initial meaning of Zuzunaga's idea. This is a way to discover those aspects of life you love, are skilled at, that you can earn money for and that others can benefit from. Then make them your choice for your career and the primary direction your life should follow.

The Great Ikigai

As we'll learn in the book you can choose two different ways of looking at Ikigai as a reference to the depth of the idea. Japanese discover Ikigai in their daily activities as well as simple pleasures. The act of brushing your child's hair can be Ikigai simply for the pleasure of it. The drive through the cookie factory while you commute to work and inhaling the fresh scent of cookie could make you feel like your favorite Ikigai. The sunset view could become your Ikigai. These are all activities that can give your life worth, even if they're not necessarily the most important thing in your life. This doesn't mean they are any less valuable or important in the quest for Ikigai.

There's a different approach to looking at Ikigai as it involves the more profound and meaningful aspects of your daily life. In the same way as the previous instance, rinsing your daughter's hair could be an obvious Ikigai but it can be a part of the deeper and more significant Ikigai. There is value to your daily life by caring for your children. This Ikigai allows you to enjoy delight in these moments, however, it's also something you are able to carry throughout the most difficult times. That's the kind Ikigai that can be used to make crucial decisions in your life , and then change it completely. The two perspectives of Ikigai are linked, they are complementary however, they're not identical.

The Purpose Venn Diagram will help to identify the second type of Ikigai that is the more profound Ikigai. This is logical since the search for a deeper significance and purpose is more prevalent across Western culture. The Japanese are looking for greater meaning and value as well however they are more accustomed to finding happiness in the smallest things than us. In western society when we think "What is the significance of our lives?"

We're typically seeking a deeper and significant answer. This is the main focus on this chart. Zuzunaga developed this idea at the time when he believed that his life was meaningless This is a typical starting point for people who find Ikigai. After experiencing this stage the artist created a sketch that was designed to assist anyone who feels like this. It's meant to help you discover an objective that can serve as the foundation for your entire existence.

Contrary to Ikigai's Venn Diagram in the same way as Ikigai

It is the most widely-known conception of Ikigai in Western culture. If you search at Ikigai through the Internet it is likely that you will come across a picture that shows Ikigai on the Purpose Venn Diagram. The diagram can be very useful, and there's no reason not to make use of it, particularly as it seems to be adapting very easily to modern life. It's not necessary to use this diagram to get to Ikigai There are plenty of exceptions to Ikigai that aren't in the framework of this diagram.

Ikigai Doesn't require payment

We've already said that Ikigai does not have to be focused on cash. There are many opportunities to use Ikigai doing things that aren't profitable or productive in any way. If you see something worthwhile in caring for your garden but it doesn't earn you any money and it's not going to help you to provide for your family or in other ways. But that doesn't mean that the Ikigai isn't worthwhile or should not be taken up. The importance of happiness is greater than money, and having an Ikigai will keep you on track and increase your productivity in other areas of your daily life. That's great enough on its own.

There are some who do encounter Ikigai at work. One of the best methods to ensure you have a good life, increase productivity and achieve success in your professional life is to discover something meaningful and valuable in the work you do for your livelihood or do things that already give you Ikigai. This is a goal every person should strive for as much as feasible. If you are at a job that you dislike because of any reason, and you've always wanted to be in a totally different field of work, consider ways to transition to your dream job gradually. The thing to remember is that just because you might have Ikigai at work does not mean all the worth in your life must be present. There is also satisfaction and meaning when you watch the television at home with the family following a long work day but that's not productive.

Ikigai Doesn't Need Proficiency

The notion that your Ikigai should be something you are skilled at is preposterous. True, you may have meaning by examining your abilities and talents. It is also possible to gain the value in using your abilities and capabilities to help others. In addition, if you realize your Ikigai is something you can consider an art and you are willing to take it seriously then you're likely to develop and master the area until it becomes one of your strengths. But, Ikigai isn't always about ability or ability, and you don't have to be an expert in something to be able to see the meaning behind it. Waiting until you're proficient enough to do something could hinder your progress and make it difficult to enjoy life to the highest degree. There is a lot to be gained from the art of drawing however, when you look at your work, it can appear like something you'd draw as a 5-year-old. You might find value in skating on ice with your spouse however, every time you go to the rink you'll spend longer on the floor than skating. There are people who are naturally poor at certain skills regardless of how they train and practice, they're not able to get better. It may sound sad however it doesn't have to be. There is no need to be a pro to be able to do it. Don't let anyone tell that you shouldn't try it simply because you don't possess the skills for it. The most tragic thing would be to be unable to live your Ikigai because you're embarrassed to try it.

The other aspects of life aren't based on skill They can also give the life a meaning and a value. There are food competitions all over the world. There is surely someone who can eat massive amounts of ice cream within five minutes. However, no one cares if you're able to do it and not observe you eating the ice cream. If your Ikigai is savoring various flavors of ice cream across the globe You don't have to be a pro to be able to do it, therefore you shouldn't bother you with it. Discover the value in your daily life, without worrying about whether you're skilled at it or not.

Ikigai Doesn't Really Need Charity

The desire to make this world more beautiful to live is an ideal goal. There's nothing wrong with directing your Ikigai towards something that can aid your community and society. It is important to think of ways to add value to your life in ways that could benefit others too. If you are looking around and feel that there are a lot of youngsters who have a low moral compass, who are in danger of falling into an addiction or commit some crime later in life It's not a bad idea to consider helping those in need. You can add value to your own life by teaching your children to play sports or play a musical instrument which is a perfectly acceptable Ikigai. In the end, the world could be a more peaceful one if we could consider what they could offer to the people in need. The problem is that we believe that Ikigai is no Ikigai without servitude. This isn't the truth.

The world can benefit from your teaching experience at a preschool or helping patients with illnesses as a nurse. However, the world doesn't require you to buy a brand new puzzle and then spend all day doing it. Finding fulfillment and joy is significant enough to allow some time for leisure. Every single thing you do should be devoted to helping others. It's important to find time to indulge yourself, without feeling guilty or shame. Ikigai isn't required to answer "what is the world really needs for me?" but that doesn't mean it's any less important.

Ikigai Doesn't Really Need Joy

This is the most debated issue, however, this is generally true in those in the Japanese population. Ikigai is usually something that brings you happiness, however it could be a thing that serves you a reason, even if you aren't a fan. Certain people are placed in positions which aren't the best however it doesn't mean that they cannot discover the significance behind them. One of the responsibilities of nurses is cleaning the bodily fluids and feces from patients in need. This is a difficult job but some nurses from Japan might find Ikigai working in this dirty work. They understand that caring for patients is messy, but it's rewarding since they understand they're in need of it. It's a noble task that they carry on their shoulders to assist others in their vicinity. Ikigai could be a shambles However, even in these instances it's still useful and significant.

This type of Ikigai not the kind of thing you should be searching for if you're looking to be content. However most people don't have this kind of life due to their own the choice of. In reality, many are caught in such situations and then find it easier to live with them because they've discovered something meaningful in these situations. If you're fortunate enough to always see Ikigai in things that you enjoy You're blessed. It could be even more fortunate to spot Ikigai in things that you dislike. If a member of your family is sick caring for them can be a hassle. But, it's clear that it's an obligation you have to take on and a duty you should not put off, and it's going to be much more enjoyable for you if you can find some value in it. Do not seek an existence that is filled with unpleasant worth. Instead, you should learn to see something valuable in the inevitability areas of your life you don't like. It's obvious that to achieve this, you need to be willing to accept that Ikigai often refers to something that you do not particularly like.

A Grounded and Occidental Philosophy

The main issue Japanese individuals will face with the diagram of Zuzunaga is the necessity of monetizing your Ikigai. Your life's purpose isn't necessarily to make money in order to be considered valid. The cultures of these societies prioritize spiritual and personal growth over the desire to make a profit. The focus on personal and emotional improvement allows us to take a an uplifting and spiritual path , resulting in greater results at the conclusion the course of life. As we age things that we own begin losing their significance, and we are forced to prioritise other aspects of our lives. In the meantime we need to find ways to put food on our tables and provide for our families. Finding an Ikigai that meets all your requirements as well as your desire for economic stability, will dramatically increase the likelihood of you being content.

Ikigai is from an era and a place when money was not so crucial. The people weren't as able to trade or prosper. Instead the Japanese were able to perform their duties and did to live (like many other civilizations at the time). This philosophy has significant connections to the time and influences the cultures of the east as well as the society. The Japanese typically view the notion of Ikigai as the search for significance and meaning within their daily lives. It's a notion that is separate from the notion of finding a significance to life and the most important factor to grow professionally. The modern world is one of freedom where you can succeed and prosper with the fruits of your labor. This is a higher priority in the current west. Western society is a place where people value professional advancement and possessions of material value more than the east. It is not necessary to rely solely on money to experience satisfaction and happiness. However working and contribute to the success of society remains important and must be taken into consideration when pursuing a pursuit of worth. In search of Ikigai in Western culture is a good reason to take into account our career goals in order that we can feel content throughout our lives.

Chapter 8: Four Feelings That Influence The Course Of Your Ikigai Discovery Journey

The four emotions have a significant impact on the ability of you to discover your ikigai, and to fulfill it in order to lead an enjoyable and fulfilling life. They are all pleasant however they can go two ways. They can aid you in finding the ikigai you've always wanted to live and enjoy. But, they may also hinder you from truly achieving your goals of ikigai. Which are the four feelings?

* Satisfaction

* Comfort

* Thrill

* Delight

Satisfaction

The feeling of satisfaction is what that you feel when you do something you enjoy and excel at, and earn money from it. It's a blend with your love for, passions, and work. If you are involved in activities you love and excel at and can earn money from, you are likely to be content with your life. Every day you leave work with a sense of satisfaction. It's not easy when the feeling gets overwhelming. However, the downside is that you could be stagnant and not be able to change.

As you've already guessed, ikigai is meant to grow over time. It is extremely likely that you'll have only one goal throughout your life. If you're too happy with your life, it can be difficult to make the necessary changes when the time is right. If your goal has changed, but you're stuck, you're likely to be in the same place you were before with a sense of happiness, satisfaction, or happiness. The most unfortunate thing is that you could be unable to connect with other people around the globe and especially with those that are important to you. Never get too satisfied. Be open to change as they occur. The trick is to find the right balance between this feeling. Make sure you aren't feeling overwhelmed, yet don't be unhappy either. What can you tell whether there's an equilibrium? As long as you are feeling satisfied after finishing your day's tasks, it indicates that you are satisfied. But, if your satisfaction increases to the point that you don't want to do anything else or go on other excursions, it means that it's getting excessive, and you must check your own level of satisfaction.

Comfort

The emotion you feel is a combination of what you excel at, what you are paid for and what people need in the world. It's what you get from your work, profession and purpose. When you make money from the area of expertise you excel in, and can utilize that skill to help others in the world, you are likely to feel at ease enough to search for the best items in your life. But, being comfortable doesn't necessarily create a meaningful life. Even if you're at ease but there is always something lacking if you're not living your ikigai to the fullest. Be aware that comfort isn't the main goal of living. Without or with the comfort of a home, life will be meaningful. But comfort doesn't matter without a purpose to the process. If you become too comfortable, you'll develop a habit of being resistant to change regardless of whether these adjustments are exactly what you require. Similar to satisfaction, the best option is to maintain a balance. Everything runs on the principle of moderation. If you are too comfortable, you could be stagnant without moving forward in your life. When people get comfortable they cease taking chances and aren't as courageous. It is because they fear losing everything they have. It's hard to live with fear in this way. If you don't feel fulfilled, your life will be dull. If you become too comfortable and do not take the initiative to change your life and passion, that's exactly what happens to you. The feeling of emptyness will always be there and tell you that you're not fulfilling your potential.

Thrill

The word "trill" is synonymous with excitement. It's the feeling that it is when you perform something you are passionate about, then give it to others and yet earn money from it. It is the result of passion, work and a mission. If you earn money through an activity that you love and are passionate about and use it to improve the lives of those to the world around you, excitement is guaranteed. You'll be looking at each day with anticipation work, instead of wishing that the workday will be over. It is the thrill that will make you want to get up each day to go to work. If there isn't enough excitement in your job it is possible to become anxious, angry and content. You might also be feeling uneasy about your capabilities. If your work doesn't inspire you and you're not happy, there's no need to do that job or the work. You should instead look for something that really thrills you. Without excitement, there'd be no reason to do it. The thrill is part of your ikigai. It's impossible to discover your passion in life and not be enthralled and thrilled. Follow whatever brings you joy. There's nothing wrong with following things you find interesting.

Delight

Delight is the feeling you feel when doing something you love or are skilled at, and are appreciated by others. It's a mix of passion, vocation and purpose. There is a deep sense of happiness that comes from connecting with other people with your work, and especially one that you are passionate about. But, regardless of the enjoyable activity but you'll struggle if it isn't making your money. Some prefer pleasure over comfort. Whatever you choose you choose, your ikigai must please you, while also earning you money, if this is what you prefer.

The secret to living a meaningful life based on ikigai is to find the right balance between the four emotions so that none of them trumps the others , or reverse. Your ikigai must be something that causes you to feel each of the four emotions when you require to feel them. The emotions, according to could affect the ability of you to achieve your ikigai when they're not in the right proportions. If your ikigai isn't generating the four feelings, living the life you want to live with meaning and meaning would be challenging. There is no meaning and satisfaction unless you're living a life that is full of joy, satisfaction, pleasure and delight. Together, these feelings create an abundance of pleasure and happiness.

What is Seken-Yoshi today?

Chapter 9: Business Model Of Making Society Happy

What are Seken-Yoshi's standards? Given our current understanding of sociology and ecology what I have come up with are the following.

Local, small, eco sustainable, socially responsible and whole-hearted.

Let me go over each the steps one by one.

Making It Small

To develop a business model that will make people happy, we have to examine our economy that is growing that was the primary obstacle standing behind.

There's no room to be found on the planet to expand. Growth doesn't necessarily mean exploring new territories anymore. It involves taking a bigger piece in the same pie. We have to figure out ways to share our resources and wealth.

According to me, circulation is key to the modern business world of the 21st century. The other word is to be content with the present situation and stop looking for more expansion. Set the limits of our growth to ensure that we share our pie with everyone who else.

It is possible to aim for enough money to feel somewhat comfortable, instead of trying to become millionaire. There's a term known as Hara Hachibunme in Japanese, meaning that you are 80% full. The phrase is commonly used when eating that we stop eating once our stomach is filled to 80. It's good for our digestive tract. Taru Wo Shiru a different expression which means to know your limit. If the goal of success is to live comfortably living, there's enough room for a lot of people to achieve success.

If you're looking to start your own business, you could begin small and consider without franchising. The 20th century saw franchising was an extremely popular model of business. Entrepreneurs would start with one location, later they'd open a second one in a different region and continue this process until they ended having a network of stores in the United States. But they didn't stop there, they expanded their business to other countries, and eventually resulted in chain stores throughout the globe.

The downside of franchise model for business is that it eliminated the possibility for locals to achieve success. For example, businesses were able to expand into new markets within their own countries and different countries. After they established franchised companies, local companies had to shut in order to avoid losing the money to compete with big firms. This made the society angry.

A small-sized business could be a good thing as you are able to focus on making the store profitable and help you lead a more enjoyable and content life since you'll have the time to develop in other aspects that you live in. Some examples are increasing your spirituality, health as well as building connections with your family and friends. This way you'll feel Ikigai throughout your life.

Making It Local

Another factor that could aid your business in achieving Seken-Yoshi's business model is to change your business's concentration from local to global.

Localizing businesses can be a part of the Seken-Yoshi model of business because it boosts locally-based economies. This is due to the fact that money circulates in communities, and this is a way to sustain the economic activity within the region in question.

Another benefit of keeping it local is that it's ecologically friendly. One of the advantages is that it stops the monoculture system of agriculture that allows farmers to plant only one crop each the year so that they can market the agricultural products. Localization facilitates the agricultural system of poly-culture , where farmers grow diverse crops to increase the diversification in the ecology.

One of the finest example of a locally-based economic system that was successful in Japan was one called a Satoyama economy.

Satoyama Economy

In Japanese the term Satoyama signifies sustainability.' Sato means livable or arable land, while the word yama refers to hills or mountains. In Japan the term Satoyama typically refers to an area that is characterized by forests, mountains, residence rice, or even vegetable fields. The reason Satoyama was a symbol of sustainability was the capacity to sustain itself by moving resources around within the area.

What happens in Satoyama can be described as the fact that the mountain ranges which are the source of rivers provide drinking water for the fields of rice and also to the houses. The village then makes use of the forests to construct homes and furniture. The removal of trees also aids in ensuring that the forest to survive since the space created was able to give way to the sunlight that young trees required to develop.

The remainder of the wood from the trees is collected along with fallen leaves. humans utilize the woods to make firewood as well as the fallen leaves to fertilize to their fields of rice. When the farmers harvest this rice out of the fields they accumulated rice bran which they can utilize as fertilizers.

As you can observe that the ecosystem was durable as each person could benefit from each other. The Japanese people practiced their Satoyama economy, which was a localized economy that relied on the flow of resources. They cultivated locally and grew a variety of food crops as they were the ones who kept the ecosystem going.

The Process of Making it Environmentally Friendly

If you make your business smaller and more localized, your business is more eco-friendly. You could also create environmentally friendly products and services that comprise organic foods, clothing made from hemp or cotton that is organically grown as well as building furniture and houses with wood from your own backyard green tourism, and more.

Making it Socially Just

One thing that was lacking in the earlier days of Japan which was a place of Satoyama economics was the notion that social justice was a concept. For instance, the work of women was more difficult than men's. Women often worked in fields alongside their husbands at work while when they came home, they were required to take care of their household chores also. Work conditions, overall was also not the best, and the majority of people had just one day off in the year. It was New Year's Day.

This is the case for Omi-merchants' ways of life also. They were away from home , leaving their wives and children behind. They spend time with their families only one month of the year. The employees were away from their homes, too, since they were recruited in Omi and then sent to work in stores in the Kanto region. They were rarely allowed to return home for the initial five years of work.

If we wish to modernize the Sanpo-Yoshi concept to modern standards ethical labor practices, ethical labour practices have to be considered.

Making It Holistic

Holistic implies that everything is connected, and when we examine things, we are looking at the whole rather than specific parts. It's similar to looking at the whole forest instead of a specific tree within it. The term is commonly used in the field medicine. In holistic medicine, doctors do not pay only to symptoms when looking at illnesses, they also consider the connections to other body organs or the patients' emotional state to see the complete picture. They don't simply prescribe medication but recommend that patients alter their habits, which are the main cause of their condition.

It is utilized in the realm of education to mean holistic education. Rudolf Steiner's Waldorf education is a wonderful illustration.

Engaging in these areas is one method of making your company more comprehensive.

Being holistic in your business isn't just about conducting business in the area of holistic education or medicine, it's also about making your working practices more whole-hearted. For instance, you would like to plan your business in a way that will allow you to spend time with family and friends. It is important to plan your business in a manner that will allow you to be in a safe and natural setting.

Through transforming the idea of Seken-Yoshi to the current standards, I feel the Sanpo-Yoshi enterprise will be the kind of Ikigai Business that is worth investing in a great deal of energy and time and will be able to feel that we're helping to advance humanity.

Chapter 10: Ikigai And Health

With an knowledge of Ikigai as well as what it's comprised of, as well as the steps to identify, define it, acknowledge it, and attain it, the next question is what exactly? Of course, having an objective in life is always rewarding however, are there any tangible advantages that come about when one finds or is on the journey to find their Igai? There are, and among these advantages is greatly better health.

Improved Mental Health

Imagine someone who has discovered their ikigai. They awake each day, and go about their routine for the day and appreciate the little things they see along the things they encounter along the. They are enthralled by the smell of their coffee, smile at their co- commuters and greet colleagues with a smile and smile and a. They start working at a slow pace, absorbed in their work. They end up

163

stopping to eat lunch with their buddies and then returning to work until it's time to go home. As they head home, they buy meals for their families, and then spend the evening with their dear families. It's a simple day, but one that many of us aren't able to see from this perspective. Anyone who has discovered their ikigai enjoys the benefits of viewing their day as this, and taking pleasure in their work as it is rather than thinking of it as work, or a chore. They are taking pleasure in their routines instead of slaving away. Imagine the benefits this will do for the mind and mental well-being.

The truth is that one doesn't need to think about it too much. One of the main causes of the growing number of depression across the globe is the constant stream of negative information that we are constantly bombarded with and feel that we're powerless and not in a position to improve our situation in life. Be aware that, before we move on, we should not believe that this concept of contentment as a sign that you should not strive to achieve greater goals, nor believe that one should not strive to make improvements in oneself. It is always a good idea to improve their own life in their surroundings and themselves, but it is the attitude one adopts that makes all the distinction. Being stuck in a rut and hating Mondays, all of these are ideas we all have heard and have been a significant factor in the decline of mental health of people all over the world in the present. Yet, appreciating our the work we do, and appreciating the things we have, instead of considering it as something we must do to survive, helps us change our perceptions and allow us to be aware the things worth living for. There are things that matter and go beyond what we initially thought of. This is the kind of thing

Ikigai can provide us with and that is the reason the reason why Ikigai is crucial to mental health.

Improved Physical Health

This is also confirmed by neuroscientific research, which shows that getting up and running on time can be beneficial to the brain. When we sleep, our brain stores the day's experiences inside our brains as well as archives and stores our memories in an absence of sensory data, which lets us reset and recharge our minds. When we wake up after we've been able to sleep enough and correctly, we wake up with our brains reenergized. Beginning the day in a positive way sets the foundation for the rest of the day. the way our brain processes the information it receives and how it is processed is crucial. Positive thinking, or at the very least a sense of contentment and acceptance reduces the amount of cortisol which is the stress hormone that gets released in our bodies throughout the day. It can be beneficial to us, because it increases our feelings and think, but has less of an impact on our bodies, since cortisol that is released in large amounts makes our body anxious and ready to respond. the stress-related "fight or fight" reaction enhancing our body's capacity to react in the moment however at the expense of our long-term health. When we're not stressed the body takes greater care and is not as stressed and results in an increased immune system better mood, as well as overall a healthier and more balanced body.

Ikigai and Kodawari

The advantages of thinking in a smaller scale

If someone thinks of Japan it is often thought about it in terms of an industrial nation that is technologically advanced rapid-paced, and extremely. They believe that it's an area where everything is work, and everything is about perfection. Most people believe that until they go to Japan and experience the country on their own. Japan is an amazing country to explore not just because of its rich culture and breathtaking natural beauty spots however, it is beautifully crafted and well-designed that tourists are amazed at how things function and how well they're taken by the staff. Many times tourists comment on how great the standard of service and how professional the presented things are and how attentive citizens are to the smallest details. From the down-to second time of trains arriving at the station, to the speedy efficient, speedy, and quick serving of a bowl of noodles at a local Ramen restaurant All of these are things that delight tourists and tourists however, they are thought to be commonplace for the Japanese. The people of Japan are accustomed to nothing less than the very best, and their standards are so high that even one or two seconds in the arrival of a train can make drivers embarrassed and warrant an public apology. What's so remarkable about this when contrasted to the majority of other nations where a delay that is one or two minutes isn't given attention to, if whatsoever?

This desire for perfection, this group and national determination to make everything as perfect as it can be is an outcome of the idea of Kodawari. Kodawari is a term that is hard to translate literal and could become literalized into English in the form of "commitment" or "insistence". But neither of these terms truly convey the meaning behind kodawari. Kodawari is typically a benchmark that people set to themselves. It is a benchmark to which one should expect to follow as closely as they are able. The majority of the time it is used to indicate the service is or how professional one is. Kodawari is a way of thinking that requires oneself to keep the highest quality in everything they do and in close proximity to that is pride, the satisfaction of taking care of everything properly, and satisfaction in the ability to achieve the standard one sets for them. In simple terms, kodawari is an approach which will take care of everything even, and in reality particularly, the smallest things. It is evident that this goes back to the initial principle of Ikigai beginning with a small amount.

If we take a take a look at Japanese culture and culture, one thing we can observe is the apex of small shops, small shops, something you would not expect in a country known for its giant industrial conglomerates. This is a tribute to the idea of ikigai and kodawari. The Japanese people are proud of doing things right. And If one stops by these small eateries and shops you will notice the attention and care given to each and every aspect, from the design and layout and the salad bowl which is served to the facilities that are offered to customers. In reality, the small neighbourhood ramen shops may be the most perfect illustration of kodawari in which restaurant owners manage their businesses because they are passionate about their job and not because they have a real goal of making money however, they have a the motivation to do everything correctly even the smallest of details, making sure that each procedure is done to perfection.

Ikigai, Kodawari, and Improving our lives

One could be wondering, how does kodawari help self-improvement? One must think about the principle of pareto, in which 20 percent of the effort results in

80 percent of the outcome. Simply put, this is the concept of diminishing returns. The longer you spend the less the benefit in comparison to the amount of time. Let's take a look at sketches. A sketcher can draw an adequate sketch within a couple of minutes, and sketches that take five minutes to complete could look very attractive. But, if the artist puts in an entire hour of work and put in a lot of effort, the quantity of detail they include will grow dramatically and the sketch will look better, but the extra time of fifty-five minutes will not produce much of a change as the initial five minute when a blank canvas or piece of paper was turned into sketches. However, those additional fifty five hours could prove to be the difference between a work that is decent and one that is outstanding. This is the place where the first pillar steps into. By putting the "just sufficient" effort to make it through and accomplishing all the

important tasks required of you it is possible to do this. But, if someone wants to get their ikigai right, they won't be content to be satisfied with "just enough" as well as "good sufficient". A greater amount of attention will be paid to the small details to enhance the overall quality of the product. A good example is in media, for instance in films or video games. What makes these games look stunning? Could it be the CGI? Perhaps it's the focus on particulars, to the extent that it is impossible to identify it as CGI where careful consideration was given to making sure that the insert was created in the most perfect way feasible, with care made to ensure that every blade of grass had real physical physics behind it. Movies and games in which these small elements are considered are incredibly immersive and consequently are lauded for outstanding work. This is what happens through starting with the smallest as the foundation of ikigai.

A good instance that is a type of kodawari that is unique to Japanese is the concept of Sembikiya. Although the idea of Sembikiya might not be a familiar concept to many, most have heard about expensive fruits, like the muskmelons or strawberries, which are available in japan. Sembikiya is a premium fruits that are grown with such concentration on detail that they're extremely expensive however, they taste higher than what you would think of from the typical fruit. The attention to precision and attention paid to the making of the fruits results in their astronomical price. They are certainly more flavorful than typical, however, take a look at the 20 thousand yen cost or more for the Sembikiya Muskmelon to just the price of a few hundred or couple of thousand yen for an ordinary one. It is possible to think that it is excessively expensive, but when one considers the attention to detail given to it during its making and processing, it could turn out at a bargain. It is after all fruit that are well taken care of that they follow the principle of one stem for single fruit production. This means that the other fruits are removed to ensure all nutrients are concentrated in the only fruit that remains. After all that effort, after all the cash spent eating it, which some say it's a wonderful experience, takes only just a few minutes. This is how kodawari is further connected to the foundations of ikigai. The present moment is the time present. The fifth pillar is about how we can reap the benefits of our efforts. Kodawari is the term used to describe paying particular attention to even the smallest detail however the results of all the work, and of the effort put into it, will last only for a short time and are regarded as fleeting.

This is evident in the Japanese pleasure of Hanami where the beauty, the ephemeral nature of the blossoms is celebrated and admired. The Japanese fascination with the beautiful and fleeting beauty can be evident in their many customs, like this. This is why they have that fifth principle of Ikigai the understanding that, even if we invest all of our time and energy to something, there will be moments when we can are able to enjoy the results of our efforts only for a short period of time and, in order to truly appreciate and appreciate it, we must be present in the moment at the present moment, in the present and now.

Conclusion

If you've made it this far, I think this book worth your time.

The two Ikigai and Kaizen Both are Japanese strategies for longevity satisfaction, happiness, and a happy life. Ikigai refers to identifying the value of your life. Kaizen refers to tiny but crucial improvement.

Ikigai can be described as the Japanese method of living that is linked with your beliefs and your purpose that ultimately refers to "the motive behind why you rise each day." Ikigai is a way of life that focuses on the "why" you Ikigai idea helps you discover the value of small things that help you live a life that is fulfilling. It's also about finding an objective that is not tied to your mind and body. Being able to adapt your actions according to your Ikigai is crucial to ensure that you have a purpose to your life, even if you transition from being an adult in your teens to becoming a parent or retiree.

Kaizen is about constant improvement through small steps to bring about more positive change. Instead of focusing on larger personal goals that seem impossible The Kaizen idea will allow you to see how you can alter your habits every day to enhance the quality and effectiveness of your activities. This will help remove the mental hurdle that often hinders you from implementing the change initially that, in turn will make the process easier to achieve and more achievable.

The book has truly addressed and the reader with various important topics that relate to the fundamental principles in Kaizen philosophy. Ikigai concept along with the Kaizen philosophy.

We talked about the Blue Zones as well as the Hara Hachi Bu diet idea. We also spoke about the five foundations of Ikigai and the four elements of Ikigai as well as physical exercises that will help you unlock your Ikigai including Radio Taiso, Yoga, Tai Chi, and Qigong.

We also talked about the beginnings and the history of Kaizen, Kaizen philosophy, four methods of Kaizen the top advantages of Kaizen and the importance of implementing Kaizen within your own life.

This brings our book to the conclusion! I am convinced the book can greatly aid you in understanding the Ikigai system and the Kaizen concept, so that you can implement them in your life in order to realize your goals of longevity, happiness and a fulfilled life GREAT success!

Thank you again for reading this Book I truly would like to wish you a very happy and prosperous future!

Thank You and best of luck!

www.ingramcontent.com/pod-product-compliance
Lightning Source LLC
Chambersburg PA
CBHW060334030426
42336CB00011B/1343